EAT CLEAN
LIVE LEAN

············••

ART GREEN'S
HEALTHY ACTION PLAN

With 35 delicious, simple paleo recipes
and 30 illustrated exercises

WITH SARAH ELL

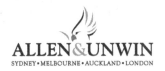

ALLEN&UNWIN
SYDNEY • MELBOURNE • AUCKLAND • LONDON

First published in 2016

Copyright © Arthur Green, 2016

Internal photographs copyright © Emerald Green Photography, 2016

Allen & Unwin
Level 3, 228 Queen Street
Auckland 1010, New Zealand
Phone: (64 9) 377 3800
Web: www.allenandunwin.co.nz
Email: info@allenandunwin.com

83 Alexander Street
Crows Nest NSW 2065, Australia
Phone:(61 2) 8425 0100

A catalogue record for this book is available
from the National Library of New Zealand

ISBN 978 1 877505 61 4

Cover photograph by Scott McAulay
Cover and internal design by Kate Barraclough
Diagram design by Janet Hunt

Printed and bound in Australia by Griffin Press

10 9 8 7 6 5 4 3 2

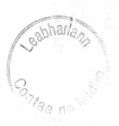

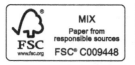

CONTENTS

· · · · · · · · · · · · · · ·•

SECTION 1: Eat Clean

Section 2: Live Lean

Section 3: Other Important Stuff

INTRODUCTION

••••••••••••••••

Hey, well done! Whether you have purchased this book, or are just flicking through it while wasting time at a bookshop, it means that you are genuinely interested in your health and wellbeing, which is a great thing in anyone's book, including mine — pun intended. Go, you!

Of course, there is the chance that you have been given this book by someone who doesn't know you well enough to know that you don't really care about any of this sort of stuff, or you might think that you are perfectly healthy just the way you are. But, if that's you, I urge you to give this book a go for at least a few more pages before you throw it in the bin or re-gift it to an uncle.

The purpose of this book is not to preach; it's not to tell you how to do things; and it's not to tell you what's right and what's wrong. It is to share with you everything I have learnt about health, nutrition, fitness and wellbeing, and to give you a bit of an insight into my life and why I consider myself to be healthy. Once you have this knowledge, it is up to you to decide if you want to apply some of this stuff to your own life in order to improve it.

This is not a foolproof plan or a rule book. The words and ideas are my beliefs about health and wellbeing, which I have developed over nearly a decade of education, research and experimentation. Once I've told you a bit about myself, this book starts out looking at optimal nutrition and gives an explanation of the paleo phenomenon — how this way of eating natural, unprocessed foods like our ancestors did has become so popular. I'll then explain what the paleo lifestyle entails — the foods I choose to eat and what I avoid — and how you can get started on it, too. There's then a section on exercise, which I think should be a critical part of all human lives: it doesn't matter how 'clean' you eat if you're spending most of your time sitting on the couch! I finish up by bringing it all together, under the heading of 'Wellbeing' — getting enough sleep, reducing stress and generally being good to yourself.

So go into this book with an open mind. Some of the information may be of use to you; some may not. You might be eager to start trying out aspects of it before you finish reading the whole thing, or you might completely skip chapters that you feel don't apply to you. And that's cool! It doesn't really matter. Read this book however you like, take from it whatever you like, but enjoy it, because it's a fun book that I believe will improve your general health and wellbeing, and most probably make you happier!

SO, WHY TAKE MY ADVICE?

•••••••••••••••

You might be thinking, 'All right, Art, I'll take a look. But, before I go any further, I want to know why should I listen to you and be taking your advice?'

Yep, good point. I had a feeling you might ask that, so I thought it would be a good idea to give you a brief background of my education and experiences, and how they led to me adopting a paleo lifestyle and becoming involved in my business, CleanPaleo. Hopefully this will give you an understanding of where I'm coming from, and why I think I can help you to lead a healthy lifestyle.

I was born in Hunterville in the Rangitikei and grew up on a small farm outside of Martinborough in the Wairarapa. Dad worked on the land, and Mum looked after me and my older sister. It was a really cool way to grow up — we didn't have a TV until after I'd started school, and I just used to spend all my time running around outside. Mum had her vege garden and my parents used to see how much we could live off the land, growing most of our fruit and veges, eating home-kill meat, getting eggs from the chooks and milk from the cow. Mum baked bread and we were all involved in doing stuff around the farm.

My parents split up when I was seven, and my sister and I moved to Wellington with Mum. Mum went back to uni and retrained in information technology, then we moved to Christchurch, where I went to Burnside High.

I was a really sporty kid at primary and high school. I was into athletics, rugby and cricket, and at high school concentrated on the javelin (I was looking for a sport where I didn't have to do any running — at that time I hated running, though I love it now).

My sister and I still spent a lot of time with Dad, and I think that's where I got my sporty genes from. Dad was always really fit and into exercise, and played representative rugby when he was younger. When I was growing up, he always had time to run around or throw a ball with me. For as long as I can remember, he's always had a home gym in the shed, built out of a few beer crates and weights made from tractor axles and drench containers! I used to go in there when I was a kid and watch him and try to 'work out' myself, using tin cans. He's still got a home gym — he might have had to replace the odd crate, but exercise is still an important part of his lifestyle.

So I guess I grew up thinking these two things were

really important for a healthy life: good-quality, natural food and regular exercise. It's the way that ideally we would all live — as close to nature as possible — though it's harder to do once you live a busy life in a city. But it was a great way to have grown up, and it's stayed with me and had a big influence on my decision to adopt a paleo lifestyle.

Once I finished school I decided to go to uni at Otago, to study exercise and sports science at the School of Physical Education. Because of my sport, I was really interested in how the body works, and I'd really enjoyed PE at high school. It was a great degree and I learnt a lot about anatomy, physiology, nutrition, psychology and the many benefits of exercise. I look back at my time at Otago as four of the best years of my life (so far!). I made some incredible friends, had a lot of fun and even found time to study.

After uni I tried a few different jobs, but hadn't really found something I wanted to do, when I got offered a job running a gym at a mining settlement in the Pilbara, a region of outback Western Australia. It was good money, and I felt it was somewhere I could actually use my degree. I could call on what I'd learnt about exercise physiology and put it into practice — even though it was in the middle of nowhere.

It was a bit of a big call, but it turned out to be one of the best decisions I ever made, because it gave me the opportunity to really look at my own health and fitness, and to discover what worked best for me. Plus I earned enough to pay off my student loan!

GETTING INTO PALEO

Towards the end of my time in the Pilbara I began throwing ideas back and forth over the ditch with a couple of mates, Ryan Kamins and Mitchell McClenaghan. Mitch is one of New Zealand's best super-good cricketers — a fast bowler — and has played for the Black Caps for the past few years, while Ryan is an incredibly bright young entrepreneur. The three of us had met about six months before I went to Australia, when we were working on the set of the US TV series *Spartacus*, which was being filmed in Auckland. (It was more fun than work, actually — we spent half our time running around sword-fighting and the rest of the time hanging out and brainstorming business ideas. What's not to like?)

Anyway, at the same time as I had been working out my own nutrition plan in Australia, these two back in New Zealand had both got into what was becoming known as 'paleo'. This is a lifestyle which basically rejects highly processed 'modern' foods and goes back to eating what our ancestors would have eaten: meat, fruit and vegetables, nuts and seeds, with no grains or processed sugars (I'll go into this in much more detail in chapter 2).

Mitch had got on to paleo after he'd had three hip operations, which had knocked him out of cricket for a while. An incredibly focused and driven individual, Mitch was not happy to just sit around and simply wait for his operations to heal; he wanted to get back on the pitch as quickly as possible, as he had the goal of playing for New Zealand firm in his sights. He decided to give a paleo lifestyle a try to drop some weight and also decrease any inflammation in his body, in the hope of accelerating his recovery. Sure enough, against all odds, just over a year after his operations Mitch got the call-up for the Black Caps, and has been taking wickets ever since. Mitch attributes his rapid recovery primarily to his change of lifestyle.

Ryan, on the other hand, had been struggling not physically but mentally. In his final year of university, for an unknown reason, Ryan's mental state went downhill. After seeing a psychologist, he was deemed to be showing symptoms of psychosis, schizophrenia, depression and anxiety. He was then referred to a neurologist and psychiatrist who sent him in for MRI scans and ECG tests on his brain. They didn't find anything in the tests, and his symptoms continued to worsen. He was now having involuntary body movements and muscle spasms as well as the mental issues. Based on these symptoms, he was diagnosed with temporal lobe epilepsy and Tourette's syndrome. He was put on medication, in an attempt to reduce his symptoms, but it didn't help and he stopped taking it after a few months.

Ryan didn't know what to do; he couldn't concentrate on his studies and began working on *Spartacus*, where he met Mitch and me. This was where Mitch told Ryan about paleo and how it was helping him. Initially, Ryan thought it was a crock and that Mitch was a dreamer, but, with few options remaining to him, Ryan bought some books on paleo and decided to give it a go. After four to six weeks following a strict paleo lifestyle, he began to feel the cyclone going on inside his head ease and become calm again. Ryan has continued with a paleo lifestyle and no longer experiences any of his symptoms to the extent that he used to.

These two had both found that this new lifestyle had dramatically improved each of their lives in different ways, and decided that they wanted to help others to improve their lives accordingly. So they had set up a company producing paleo foods, such as breakfast cereals, protein powders and snacks, for people who wanted to adopt a paleo lifestyle but were lacking the time to make everything from scratch.

CleanPaleo had been up and running for just under a year when they asked me if I wanted to come on board, and my answer was a big yes! Finally I'd found something which brought together what I'd learnt at uni and during my time at the mine, something that I really believed in and that I thought could help other people too. Winning!

And of course there's that other thing I should really mention . . . *The Bachelor*. Being on that show was an incredible experience. It ended up working out better than I could have hoped, and has presented me with a lot of opportunities. And what does that have to do with my lifestyle? Well, in all honesty, do you think I would have been asked to be the bachelor if I hadn't made a conscious effort to keep myself muscular and lean? I'll talk some more about society's expectations later (see pages 252-254), but let's just say for now that they exist and you might as well use them to your advantage.

So that's how I got to where I am today: living a paleo lifestyle and helping other people to enjoy its benefits. But don't just take my word for it — you need to try for yourself. Get reading and experimenting, and I'm pretty sure it won't be long before you start to see and feel the benefits.

Cool. Let's kick on with it, shall we?

SECTION I
EAT CLEAN

1. WHY IS WHAT I EAT SO IMPORTANT?

················•

'There are so many different diets and eating guidelines, some of them conflicting. It's confusing and makes it impossible to know what I should be eating. One day I'm told that I should be eating one thing, and the next day I'm told that it's going to make me fat and I should be eating something else.' Ever felt like this? It does your head in! And now you've picked up this book hoping it's going to contain the one true answer . . .

Well, not quite. Unfortunately I don't think any book or any person is able to do that, because I don't believe that there is one true answer to optimal nutrition — at least, not one that applies to everyone. Instead, I'm going to share with you what I believe the ideal diet for the human body is based on everything I've learnt and everything I've experienced.

I think the key to finding the best nutritional regime for your body is to educate yourself as much as possible about the different options, and to try things for yourself to determine what works best for your body and makes you feel great. Luckily for you, I have spent years doing this and so, by reading this book, you can save a bit of time! (See chapter 3 for more on my journey.) I will explain why I think some things are of benefit, because most of what I have found out about food and how our body processes it is very interesting. Armed with this knowledge, you will be able to make up your own mind about what you should eat.

Firstly, in order to explain why I don't believe there is only one answer to optimal nutrition, let's take a look at what nutrition actually means. And I don't mean that in a figurative way; I mean let's *literally* look at the definition of the word according to the *Oxford Dictionary* online (oxforddictionaries.com):

nutrition
noun
1. the process of providing or obtaining the food necessary for health and growth.
2. the branch of science that deals with nutrients and nutrition, particularly in humans.

OK, cool. So this tells us that nutrition has a couple of meanings: firstly, it is the process of eating food to help us be healthy and grow; and, secondly, it is a science that looks at that food and how it affects the body from a biological and physiological point of view.

So, if nutrition is a science, you'd think there should be some clear-cut facts about what is good for us and what is bad for us, and therefore what is the right diet and what is the wrong diet for us. Right? Wrong. Well, at least, I don't believe it's as easy as that. Yes, countless studies have been performed to determine how different foods affect us biologically, and these studies provide us with solid, factual information. The problem is that the human body is so unbelievably complex that, while one thing might indeed be good for us in one way, in another way it might actually be harmful. You can find this simply by having a google: if you can find a study that says one food is beneficial, you can probably search again and get a list of studies stating the negative effects of the same thing.

What scientists think is good or bad for us changes over time, too. When the US Department of Agriculture published its first healthy diet recommendations in 1894, what we know today as the key vitamins had not even been discovered. The traditional Western diet that most of us have been brought up with and had drilled into us at school is the Food Pyramid. The US Department of Agriculture came up with this in the early 1990s and you're probably familiar with its message: lots of bread, rice, cereals and pasta, plenty of fruit and vege, a bit of dairy, meat, eggs and a little bit of fats, oils and added sugars at the top.

A TRADITIONAL FOOD PYRAMID

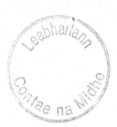

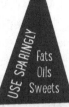

USE SPARINGLY

Fats
Oils
Sweets

Milk
Yoghurt
Cheese

2-3
SERVINGS

Meat
Poultry
Fish
Dry beans
Eggs
Nuts

2-3
SERVINGS

Vegetables

3-5
SERVINGS

Fruit

2-4
SERVINGS

Bread, cereal, rice & pasta

6-11
SERVINGS

Fats got a bad rap from the 1950s, when an American doctor named Ancel Keys published a study of the causes of coronary heart disease in seven countries. He pointed the finger firmly at dietary fat for causing cholesterol build-up, cherry-picking data from seven countries out of a possible 22 to support his hypothesis. He must have made his study sound pretty convincing, because scientists, doctors and government health bodies around the world took his word for it and all of a sudden fats — especially animal fats like those found in meat and animal products like butter — were the devil's work and we were all going to die of clogged arteries quick smart if we didn't lay off! As you can imagine, this made Keys pretty unpopular with the meat and dairy industry. Nevertheless, this anti-fat mantra became widely accepted. The unfortunate side effect of this was that food manufacturers, responding to pressure from governments and the public to reduce the fat content of their products, started to fill them up with other things to keep them tasting good: nasties like sugar and salt. What followed was a gradual increase in obsesity levels and rates of diseases relating to bad diet, among them Type 2 diabetes and heart disease.

By the 2000s, the traditional healthy eating pyramid had been discounted, and Harvard Medical School came up with its own pyramid, which placed daily exercise and weight control on the bottom, plus plenty of vegetables and fruits, healthy oils, nuts and seeds, fish, poultry and eggs. A step in the right direction, but this pyramid also suggested eating red meat

THE HEALTHY EATING PYRAMID

Dept of Nutrition,
Harvard School of Public Health

USE SPARINGLY

Red meat, processed meat
Butter
Refined grains (white rice,
bread & pasta)
Potatoes
Sugary drinks, sweets
Salt

OPTIONAL

Alcohol in moderation
(not for everyone)

Dairy (1-2 servings/
day) or vitamin D/
calcium supplements

FOR MOST PEOPLE

Daily multivitamin
plus extra vitamin D

Nuts, seeds,
beans & tofu

Fish,
poultry
& eggs

Vegetables
&
fruits

Healthy
fats/oils

Whole
grains

Daily exercise & weight control

23

sparingly, and keeping wholegrains in there as a staple. As you will read in the next chapter, I believe we can go a step further in defining the optimum nutritional regime for human beings. I also believe that within the next ten years we are going to see that healthy eating pyramid revised again, as science catches up with what thousands of people around the world are experiencing by adopting a paleo lifestyle.

WHY WE EAT

I think a question that's just as big as 'what should I eat' is 'why do I eat'? In our society, eating food is more than just a matter of meeting our nutritional needs, otherwise we'd all just be able to drink some ideal nutritional concoction three times a day and save ourselves a lot of time — and dishes.

For most of us, eating is a social act. Most of the time we eat in the company of others, whether it's breakfast with flatmates, lunch in the lunchroom or at a café with colleagues, or dinner with friends and family. Eating provides breaks in the day, a chance to have a pause and refuel emotionally as well as physically. But, unfortunately, these social aspects can have a negative effect on us if we're trying to watch what we eat and take care of ourselves. It's much harder to not have a piece of cake to celebrate a birthday at work if everyone else in the office is having one; you get in trouble if you tell your mother that no, you won't have a second helping of her delicious lasagne; and it's hard not to snack on chocolate when your flatmates are sitting around scoffing it while you watch TV together. Some studies have also shown that we tend to eat more when we eat with other people than when we eat alone.

And, of course, we eat because we enjoy it. Food is delicious! (Or it should be, otherwise you need to learn to cook better!) We all have our favourites, whether crispy bacon, a tender steak, smooth ice cream, crunchy apples . . . you get the picture. And do you notice one other thing about that list? It's not just about the taste of the food; it's about texture, how the food feels as you eat it. That's one reason why I don't think real food will ever be replaced by sciency drinks or 'food pills' like something out of a sci-fi comic.

Not only does food taste good, but eating feels good. It gives us pleasure. It's one of the things that's unique to humans: we eat because we like to, not just because we need to. As long as we've eaten something reasonably healthy, our sense of being hungry goes away and we feel full (a sensation known as satiety). But it goes beyond that. Often after we've eaten certain foods we get a sense of wellbeing that is about more than not being hungry any more. This is another important aspect of why we eat — and how mindful we need to be of what we are putting in our mouths.

Many people associate emotions with something spiritual — that they just naturally spring into our brains in reaction to events and experiences — but in fact many of the emotions we experience are actually biochemical, meaning that we 'feel' certain ways due to the presence or absence of various chemicals in our brain. The big ones are endorphins: feel-good chemicals which act like opiates, blocking the brain's perception of pain. Plus there are other chemicals like dopamine and serotonin, which have important effects on our brain chemistry and therefore what we experience as emotions.

Different foods trigger different chemical responses in our bodies. Chocolate and endorphins is the most commonly known: you eat a couple of pieces of chocolate, experience the rich, sweet taste and the creamy texture on your tongue, and suddenly a flood of endorphins is released into your brain, making you feel great. (Exercise has similar effects — see pages 233–235 for more about the effects of exercise on your brain chemistry.) On the flip side, a lack of the right chemicals can have negative effects, such as depression caused by low serotonin levels.

So, when you are thinking about what you eat and what your ideal nutrition plan would be, you need to take these emotional, social and neurological factors into account. But, remember, when it comes down to it you are in control of what you eat, and it is up to you to make the best possible choices for your body.

If you are going to adopt a paleo lifestyle, it needs to be something you enjoy and feel good about. There is no point in trying to do something that you think is 'good for you' if you just feel unhappy, anxious and consumed by it all the time. You need to be able to still eat foods you enjoy without worrying about the negative effects they are having on your body, and to be able to live 'normally' in the world, not cutting yourself off from friends and family or becoming the guy no one wants to ask out anywhere because your eating regime is so inflexible and downright weird that it's too much hard work. You don't want to have to stop seeing other people or doing things you enjoy because of your 'diet'. And, most of all, you don't want to find yourself thinking, 'Man, this is waaaaay too hard. I'm just going to go back to chips and burgers and be done with it.'

The good news is, I believe the paleo lifestyle enables you to still eat foods you enjoy, never leaves you feeling hungry or unsatisfied, and you'll still be able to hang out with your mates without being 'the paleo guy/girl'. So let's find out some more about what 'paleo' means, and how it became popular.

2. WHAT IS PALEO, ANYWAY?

Say the word 'paleo', and people react in different ways. Some say, 'Isn't that the caveman diet?' Some say, 'Isn't that like a cult?' And others just say, 'That's weird, you're weird, you weirdo.'

'Paleo' is short for paleolithic, which refers to the time in human evolution when we were hunter-gatherers. The word comes from the Greek words *palaios*, meaning old, and *lithos*, meaning stone, so basically we are talking the Stone Age. This period is defined as starting about 2.6 million years ago, when human-like apes first began using stone tools, and runs until about 10,000 years ago, when humans moved to an agriculture-based lifestyle, growing crops and raising domesticated animals. So the paleo lifestyle basically means eating the same way our ancestors did, before we invented farming and when we

THE WORST MISTAKE IN THE HISTORY OF THE HUMAN RACE

Tellingly, in an article published back in 1987, evolutionary biologist Dr Jared Diamond described the adoption of agriculture by early man as 'the worst mistake in the history of the human race'. Diamond said that agriculture caused the human diet to become dependent on a handful of starchy crops of limited nutritional value, which not only reduced overall nutritional aspects but also put communities at risk of starvation if a crop failed. Taking it a step further, he argues that the social changes caused by reliance on agriculture encouraged people to live together in greater concentrations, increasing the risk of disease and creating class and power divisions. He writes, 'Hunter-gatherers practiced the most successful and longest-lasting life style in human history. In contrast, we're still struggling with the mess into which agriculture has tumbled us, and it's unclear whether we can solve it.' Whether or not you agree with Diamond's views, he does shine the spotlight on some interesting social implications caused by the development of agriculture.

had to find all our own food by hunting and foraging.

The Hollywood-generated image that springs to mind when talking about paleo is of hairy cavemen running around in animal skins, dragging sabretooth tigers back to the cave for their scantily clad women to roast over the fire, communicating in grunts. But in fact there was a huge diversity of human life during the Paleolithic period, as populations grew and spread from their origins in Africa north into Europe and east into Asia, and across land bridges into North and South America. And these people, over such an enormous period of time, obviously ate a huge and varied range of foods. But we know for sure that they didn't eat grains, which didn't become part of the human diet until agriculture became widely established at the end of the last Ice Age (when a big bout of global warming changed both growing conditions and the habitats of big game like woolly mammoths), and they certainly didn't eat processed sugar.

WHAT IS THE PALEO DIET?

The term 'the Paleo Diet' was coined by an American doctor called Loren Cordain, who first published a book with that name back in 2002. Cordain, who is now a guru of strict paleo, says he didn't come up with the diet; in the introduction to his book (of which more than 200,000 copies have been sold, not to mention all the hits on his website thepaleodiet.com) he says he 'simply uncovered what was already there: the diet to which our species is genetically adapted'.

While the book sold OK at first, it really took off in around 2010, when it started to gain popularity among

PALEO IS ACTUALLY
OLD NEWS TO NEW ZEALAND
~~~~

It's interesting to think that the diet of Maori in New Zealand before European settlers began to arrive in the early 1800s (and continuing for some time after that in areas away from missionary settlements) could be considered 'paleo'. Maori were largely a hunter-gatherer society, relying on seafood, eggs, birds such as moa, and seals for their protein intake, supplemented with plant-based foods such as kumara, taro, berries and fern roots. Captain James Cook described the people he encountered in 1769–70 as 'a strong, well-made, active people, rather above the common size'.

In 2010, nutritionist Ben Warren worked with former All Black captain Taine Randell to run a programme at Te Aranga Marae in Hawke's Bay, in which participants ate a diet based on traditional (pre-European contact) Maori foods: meat, seafood, some fats and vegetables. Significantly, over ten weeks the 27 participants lost an average of 8.7 kilograms, as well as experiencing stabilised blood-sugar levels, with many moving out of the Type 2 diabetes danger zone. Māori Television also filmed a series called *The Native Diet* in 2012, in which Maori were encouraged to eat and be active like their tupuna (ancestors) to improve their health.

the fitness community, especially people who were into CrossFit (for more on CrossFit, see page 247). Since then Dr Cordain's work and the concept of the paleo diet have become much more mainstream, and are increasingly talked about in the media and, of course, all over the internet. His view of paleo being a diet which humans are genetically adapted to eat is one I share and is the major reason why I eat this way.

Another paleo enthusiast I really respect is Robb Wolf, an American who used to be a biochemist and became a strength and conditioning coach. His book *The Paleo Solution: The Original Human Diet* (2010) is one of the first books I read about paleo, and remains one of my favourites.

So, paleo is big in the States — and getting bigger — but it's also gaining traction down under. Australian personal trainers Luke Hines and Scott Gooding off the TV series *My Kitchen Rules* have become a voice for paleo over the ditch, as has celebrity chef Pete Evans, who has become known as 'Paleo Pete' (and attracted some controversy for it). And more and more people in New Zealand are becoming interested in the paleo way of life — as evidenced by the success and growth of the company I part-own, CleanPaleo.

DIET OR LIFESTYLE?

You can read more about how I got into paleo myself in the next chapter. But, before I go on, I'd like to clarify

PALEO AT A GLANCE

WHAT IS PALEO?

When you live a paleo lifestyle, you're basically eating the same way your ancestors did, back when we had to find all our own food by hunting and foraging, before we invented farming.

WHY STEP BACK IN TIME?

The agricultural revolution turned us from hunter-gatherers to farmers. Modern Western diets are now more reliant than ever on cereal grains and their by-products. The problem is, our bodies have not had time to evolve to cope with this, so we're seeing soaring rates of obesity, Type 2 diabetes and other diet-related conditions.

FILL YOUR PALEO PLATE WITH . . .

Red meat, poultry, eggs and fish — where possible, make sure your meat is organic, free range, grass-fed and/or sustainably sourced. The closer to nature the food you eat is, the better it is for you.

Go for gold with veges — just leave out the potatoes (which are generally avoided as part of a paleo diet) and beans and peas (which contain nasties that cause yucky things like gut inflammation).

Fruit — just keep it to around two pieces a day, as it contains natural sugar. Eat seasonally and locally where

you can. Leave out the dried fruit and juice, though —
you wouldn't eat five oranges in one go, so don't do it in
liquid form either!

Nuts and seeds — high in good fats (unsaturated fats
and omega-3 fatty acids), these make great snacks and
additions to salads. Forget peanuts though; they're not
even a nut (see page 70).

SAY GOODBYE TO . . .

→ Cereal grains
→ Refined sugar
→ Highly processed foods containing additives,
   preservatives and artificial flavourings
→ Dairy products
→ Beans, peas and legumes

WHY BOTHER?

The results speak for themselves: you'll enjoy increased
energy, be less likely to get sick, and you'll be filled with
a general feeling of wellbeing and health! Who wouldn't
want that?

something: I personally like to think of and refer to
paleo as more of a lifestyle than a diet. Again, with the
Oxford Dictionary online, diet is defined as:

1. the kinds of food that a person,
   animal, or community habitually eats.

2. a special course of food to which a
   person restricts themselves, either to
   lose weight or for medical reasons.

Yes, paleo is my diet in terms of the first definition of the word, but the second definition is what scares people away. The idea of 'being on a diet' has a lot of negative connotations — starving yourself, restricting what you eat, being banned from eating things you like and so on.

For me, paleo is not like that. If you're eating 'normally' (as in, you're not on a diet) then you just eat the foods you want to eat. I want to follow the paleo template of nutrition because it's food I enjoy and know is the healthiest for me. So I'm not following a diet; I've just made the paleo template my 'normal'. Sure, there are foods which I avoid eating (more on that shortly), but mostly they are foods I don't want to eat anyway, because I know the effects they will have on my body. But I'm not counting calories or trying to eat less in order to lose weight. Paleo is a guideline, a template for which foods are best for my body and which ones I should stay away from.

I refer to paleo as a lifestyle because the way you eat changes the way you live. To eat this way, you are going to have to cook more and rely less on pre-prepared foods and takeaways (sorry!). But in return you'll feel healthier, more energetic and more positive. It'll make you want to exercise and just improve your whole lifestyle.

I don't know a single person who has tried living a

paleo lifestyle and not agreed that it is most probably the best nutritional regime for their body. I urge everyone who cares enough about their health to educate themselves as much as possible about paleo and to try it for themselves.

If you're thinking about whether or not to try paleo, I say just give it a go. It's not that scary! If it doesn't work for you, then, oh well, try something else, but don't count it out until you've tried it.

I'll give anything a go once. I gave paleo a go and just never stopped.

IS PALEO FOR EVERYONE?

I believe the paleo template is for everyone, perhaps just with varying degrees of adherence to suit a person's body and lifestyle. Every person's body is different and responds differently to different ways of eating, but I believe the paleo template is the best nutritional programme for everyone to follow. You can adapt it, individualise it and adjust it to suit your own lifestyle, however you see fit. But, by following the basic template, you will see the benefits.

It's not just for gym junkies and people who want to lose weight. In fact, if you're really into the gym and want to bulk up, paleo might not be for you — at least not in its strictest form. You're probably going to need to eat a few more carbs, which, if obtained from grains, kind of goes against the paleo philosophy. But if you want to be lean and healthy then it's definitely worth trying.

Paleo is for ordinary people who want to feel better and improve their overall quality of life. So isn't that everyone, really?

If you have any concerns at all, talk to your doctor before making any major changes to your nutrition intake.

PALEO FOR PARENTS

There was a frightening story in the media recently about children as young as three years old having their teeth extracted because they were rotten from drinking so much Coke and other sugary drinks like orange juice. Now, those kids weren't walking down to the dairy and getting that themselves — their parents were feeding it to them, in a sipper bottle!

You might think, 'Well, I'm not that kind of parent,' but think about what you are feeding your kids. Biscuits, flavoured yoghurts, juice, so-called 'healthy' snacks like muesli bars? There's a lot of sugar in that stuff, and not much else in the way of nutrition. (And I think about my own flirtation with Coca-Cola! See page 93.)

I'm not necessarily suggesting turning your kids paleo — god knows Pete Evans has got in enough trouble — but I do think you should try to make the best possible food choices on behalf of your kids. After all, you're the parent; you do have control over what food is in the house and what is served at mealtimes. Set a good example and show your kids your own healthy lifestyle choices in action. If you don't have unhealthy food in the house, they're going to find it much harder to get hold of (and teenagers are notoriously lazy — if it's not in the cupboard or fridge at home, they're not that likely to go out foraging for it).

You don't want to give your kids food hang-ups and make life hard for them — growing up is tough enough without getting shit from other kids about the weird food you eat — but give them healthy choices and show them the benefits of eating foods which are good for their bodies.

You may also find that you are able to actually see a change in your child's behaviour just by giving them healthier foods. For example, some aspects of your child's behaviour that you consider normal, such as mood swings, hyperactivity, trouble concentrating or tiredness, may be improved simply by reducing the amount of sugary food and grains that they're eating.

3. HOW I GOT INTO PALEO

You might be wondering why I started living a paleo lifestyle. Am I some kind of freak with an extreme eating regime who spends all my time in the gym? Well, I don't think so. And, while I often get labelled with the 'paleo' thing, the way I live isn't actually hard-core paleo. It's a sustainable, enjoyable way of eating that I believe meets my nutritional needs, gives me lots of energy and basically makes me feel great! Let me explain how I got into it in the first place.

I've already mentioned that I spent some time working in a mining settlement in Western Australia after I finished uni. That was where I really started to do some research on what might be the best way to eat — using myself as a guinea pig.

The Pilbara is a 90-minute flight north of Perth;

it's a large, dry, thinly populated region in the north of Western Australia. It is known for its Aboriginal peoples, its ancient landscapes, the red earth and its vast mineral deposits. It's these mineral deposits that are the reason for all of the small mining towns and camps that dot the vast, empty redness. Mining camps like these are set up for the workers, who fly in, work for a number of weeks (I would work for four weeks at a time), then fly home for a week's break before doing it all again. Living like that is not something you can do long-term — I lasted eighteen months, but that was more than enough for me. You're away from your friends, your social life, normal society — just you and a thousand other guys out in the middle of the red desert.

My camp had everything the miners needed — housing, bars and a gym. That last part was my job. Most of the miners spent their spare time in the bar but it was my role to look after the ones who wanted to be healthy and happy. (In saying that, I did manage to convert some of the bar-goers to become gym-goers; but that was a small handful — like the hand of a two-year-old child.)

At the beginning I found it pretty weird being totally isolated from the 'real world'. I had a lot of time to myself, as the miners were away working during the day and mostly only came to the gym in the evenings. I'd spend my days cleaning the gym, exercising, reading and learning . . . it was a pretty strange situation, but actually quite nice in a way. The complete opposite to my life now, that's for sure!

But after a while I started to see this as a great

opportunity for self-development. I developed a goal to become as healthy as I possibly could be. But there were so many different theories about how to be 'healthy': so many different diets, so many different forms of exercise, and so many ways to alter your mental health. So I figured that the only way to know what would be best for me personally was to try a bunch of these things out for myself.

While I'd always been into sport and exercise, I hadn't ever put much effort into my nutrition. I've always been . . . not skinny, exactly, but slim, so I'd never thought much about what I was eating. But the more I read and researched the more I realised health isn't just about weight management, but a lot more about your energy, how you feel and your mental and general wellbeing.

All the guys at the gym were always asking me what they should be eating, so I decided to have a play around and experiment on myself to figure out what worked best. I decided to use each four-week block at the mine to trial different eating regimes.

VEGETARIANISM

I started off with vegetarianism — and, trust me, this isn't easy when you are living in a camp with a thousand meat-eating miners! There was one other vegetarian in the camp, an Indian guy. He and I used to stand patiently to the side of the dinner buffet (me salivating over the steaks and chicken), waiting for the chefs to bring out the vegetarian options. At least there was always plenty of fruit to snack on.

I find the philosophy behind vegetarianism quite interesting. There are so many reasons why people choose not to eat meat. Some people don't eat meat for religious reasons. Some feel that their health will benefit from eating more fruit and vegetables and no meat. Others have made the switch to vegetarianism because they see it as more environmentally sustainable or because they are ethically opposed to eating animals. Arguably, that last point is actually pretty widely shared, even by meat-eaters: put it this way, nobody *wants* to see animals suffer. All other things being equal, given the option between killing a pig and not killing a pig, many people would choose not to kill the pig. It's when personal incentives come into play — whether those incentives are the delicious taste of bacon, or money or whatever — that people can then make a conscious decision as to whether or not the death of that animal is worth the bacon on their plate. (Mmmm, bacon . . .)

Anyway, back to my vegetarian experience. My initial thoughts were that I was not going to get enough protein in my diet to enable me to train effectively, or recover from exercise quickly enough. I took a whey-powder supplement to counteract this.

Over the course of the month I didn't notice any drastic changes to my body composition or my energy levels. I found that I could exercise at exactly the same intensity and my recovery was the same. I did find, however, that I was having to eat more food more frequently, as the fruit and vegetables that I predominantly ate did not fill me up as much as meat did. I also realised that I really missed the taste and texture of meat, and meals containing meat.

This was the first time that I realised there was more to a healthy diet than just the nutritional aspect of the food — the mental and social aspects of it were just as important. It made me realise that I could never follow a strict vegetarian diet, even if I did notice huge health benefits, as it is not sustainable for me personally or socially. So I celebrated the end of my vegetarian month with a huge T-bone steak and thought about what I would try next.

LOW CARB, HIGH PROTEIN

Next I tried a very low-carbohydrate, high-fat and high-protein diet, often referred to as a ketogenic diet (the much-discussed Atkins Diet uses some ketogenic principles). Some of the gym-goers at the Pilbara were interested in this form of diet because of its ability to make you lose body fat. I'll describe how this happens by explaining what a ketogenic diet and ketosis are.

Ketosis is essentially a metabolic state in which the body primarily relies on fat for energy. Biologically, the human body is a very adaptable machine, which can run on a variety of different fuels. On a standard, carbohydrate-heavy, Western-type diet, the primary source of energy is glucose (glucose is the energy that comes from carbohydrates when they are broken down). If glucose is available, the body will use it first, as it's the quickest substance to metabolise. So, on the standard Western diet, your metabolism will be primarily geared towards burning carbohydrates (or glucose) for fuel.

However, if there is very little carbohydrate in the diet, the liver converts fat into fatty acids and ketone bodies. The ketone bodies pass into the brain and replace glucose as an energy source. Hence the name 'ketogenic' diet. You basically just stop eating carbs, and eat fat to burn fat.

So, how did it go for me? Well, I did find that I lost body fat, and also maintained muscle mass, so it was very successful from an aesthetic point of view. I also found that my energy levels were slightly higher than normal. I did find, however, that I wasn't able to exercise at the same intensity — I was doing a lot of high-intensity cardio exercise and found that I just couldn't go as hard for as long as normal. And, although I didn't really notice anything that would make me think, 'I'm not getting the nutrients my body needs,' I couldn't help but feel that this might be the case. I think that if I had carried on not eating nutrient-rich vegetables and fruits (which contain carbohydrates) I probably would have seen some effects of nutrient deficiency after an extended period on a ketogenic diet.

ISAGENIX

The next thing I tried was Isagenix, a system of supplements and products designed for weight loss and overall health improvement. Again, a lot of people at the gym were asking me about Isagenix and, with very little reliable information on the internet about it, I decided to give it a good crack — not to lose weight, but to find out for myself what all the fuss was about and to see if it improved my energy levels.

In a nutshell, it's a nutritional supplementation regime that provides a variety of whey-protein shakes, bars and herbal supplements that promise to help you lose weight. And, rather than using traditional forms of advertising and selling, Isagenix uses multi-level network marketing, which relies on participants setting up distribution networks — basically selling to their friends. The company then pays them commissions based on sales.

There are definitely plenty of people who happily sing the praises of the programme, but I don't believe it is as great as everyone makes it out to be. One thing to remember is that no one using Isagenix is going to give you an objective testimonial, because they all have a vested interest. Basically, if they tell you it's great — and, don't get me wrong, it may well be great for them — and then you decide to start using it because of them, they can potentially make money. Just to be clear, this is not a pyramid-selling scheme; it is called network marketing or direct selling, which can be very effective. You might not like that idea, but don't judge the brand and products by its sales strategy; judge it instead on its nutritional merit, which is what I did.

I tried what they call the President's Pak, for 30 days. Long story short: I didn't really feel any different. I still needed a coffee hit to get me going in the morning, and I wasn't filled with amazing energy like I had hoped I would be. And it also made me realise that you can't beat eating real food.

I know that it has changed many people's lives for the better and I believe the system has the potential to help people who primarily want to lose weight. However, in saying this, I wouldn't recommend Isagenix to anyone who has access to a supermarket. I don't think real food should ever be replaced by supplements. By eating real food, you are getting vital nutrients, vitamins and minerals that you would never be able to get out of a packet or a container. Real food doesn't contain chemicals, additives, preservatives or anything processed that can negatively affect your body, and by eating real food you can reach your health goals just as quickly and easily. (For more on processed foods to watch out for, see page 84.)

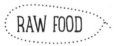

RAW FOOD

After living on supplements for four weeks, I decided to go back to basics and try a raw-food diet. For this I took a trip to Byron Bay, which is renowned for its chilled vibe, surf beaches and its fresh organic produce. While there I stayed with a friend who'd been living on a raw-food diet for a while. She showed me so many tips and tricks that made eating a raw-food diet enjoyable and far more delicious than I thought it could be. It really opened my mind to trying new things and questioning everything that I had learnt growing up regarding food. Simple foods became delicious, like eating corn on the cob raw — it was amazing! (If you haven't tried this before, I urge you next time you eat corn not to cook it. Just eat it raw and taste how sweet and juicy it is!) It was summertime so there were lots of fruits and vegetables available and we ate amazing salads every day. I definitely felt lighter — I didn't lose any weight but I just felt less stodgy and that I had more energy.

There were lots of things I really liked about eating a raw-food diet — but there were foods I missed, too. Red meat, chicken, fish and eggs were the main ones — primarily because I really enjoy eating them, but also for their nutritional value, as they are great sources of protein. Without these sources of protein in my diet, I had to rely on a protein-powder supplement to ensure that I was getting enough protein to maintain and repair my muscles as I exercised. The only two types of raw protein powder I could find were either pea or rice protein. I didn't really like either, as I found they had a chalky texture, but went with a rice protein as it has a higher biological value (BV) than pea protein — meaning more of that protein is actually used by the body (for more on protein powders and BV see chapter 11).

Another aspect of a raw-food diet becoming more prevalent is the different raw-food creations on offer at speciality cafés and restaurants. These creations are where common and staple cooked foods are created out of raw food, like raw 'nachos', 'cheesecake' or 'pizza'. These things take a lot of time to make and can be expensive — and it seems a bit unnecessary to me.

I also got a bit frustrated with the way that raw food is made out to be synonymous with healthy eating, but there are lots of recipes for and raw-food cafés that serve sweet treats which, to be honest, are not that much better for you than the non-raw versions. Even though their ingredients are more natural, these sweet treats still contain a lot of sugar and should not be overconsumed. Plus, there is a lot of food substitution that goes on — using raw-food versions of basic ingredients, such as cheese made from cashew nuts. I personally don't have a problem with the normal, natural versions of these foods and just think, 'What's the point in trying to create them out of something else?'

Again, there were things I liked about a raw-food regime, but it was way too hard to maintain once I was back at the mining camp, and would isolate me socially if I were to follow it today.

TRYING PALEO

The next step was trying a paleo diet, which combined some aspects of most of the eating regimes I had tried — some raw foods, no processed food, lots of veges and plenty of healthy protein. (You can read more about the origins of the paleo diet on page 28, and about what you should eat and should avoid in chapters 4 and 5.) I'd heard of paleo about a year before, as it was starting to become more mainstream and be talked about online and in the fitness community, and I knew Ryan and Mitch had tried it. But before then I hadn't really thought that its benefits would apply to me, as I thought it was more of a weight-loss diet.

I started to read up about it, and the more I read the more I wanted to try it. I was really interested in the philosophy behind it — the idea that this was the food our bodies were supposed to digest and the food they function the best on. It made a lot of sense to me, the idea that our bodies are not designed to eat the processed foods and farmed carbohydrates that many of us live on today — we haven't had enough time to evolve to be able to cope with them. And a paleo diet allowed me to eat the foods I liked, so I thought I'd give it a go.

I started following the paleo guidelines as strictly as possible. It really wasn't the drastic change that I thought it would be. I just stuck to meat, veges, fruits, nuts, seeds and eggs. The big thing was avoiding any grains, processed foods or anything artificial, like margarine and especially processed sugar.

I started with one of my four-week blocks, and it was like a light had been switched on. It was easy to follow and I felt great. I began sleeping better, and woke up in the mornings feeling rested and alert, rather than groggy and reaching for a coffee. There was a wide range of foods I could eat. It gave me the energy I needed to exercise at the intensity I wanted, and I recovered well from training. Finally I had found a lifestyle that worked for me. After the other diets I'd tried, this was the first regime that seemed sustainable.

With all of my other diet 'experiments', when I got to the end of the four weeks I was amping to get back to eating 'normally', and would spend my week off in the real world eating whatever I felt like. After finishing my first four-week block of paleo, when it came to my week off I found I just wanted to go on eating this way. I went back to the camp and carried on doing it. And I've been eating this way pretty much ever since. I truly believe it's the best nutritional template for the human body.

One of the biggest things about living a paleo lifestyle for me has been that I just don't seem to get sick any more. Every now and then I get the start of a cold, but it never takes hold. I used to get the flu at least once a year, but since I started eating paleo I haven't had it at all (touch wood!). There is lots of research to show that living a paleo lifestyle has hugely positive benefits to your overall wellbeing through helping to regulate the hormones in the body and improving your gut health (see page 98) and I have certainly felt the benefits of that.

I always consider myself to be 'paleo'. However, some traditionalists who are strictly paleo may argue against this, because, as you'll find out later in the book, I don't stick to it 100 per cent — I do have some dairy, and I have a beer every now and then, and I've certainly been known to eat the odd almond croissant. I like going out for a meal sometimes without having to think about what I can and can't eat . . . So maybe I'm not strictly 'paleo' — maybe I just have a healthy diet! But 'healthy' means so many different things to different people. To me, healthy means paleo, so let's use paleo for now.

'All right, Art,' you might be saying. 'Enough of the chit-chat. I need to know the facts. What foods am I allowed to eat, seeing as woolly mammoth is in short supply in Ponsonby? What foods are definitely out?'

Well, let's have a look at what you should and shouldn't eat, and why people who have a paleo lifestyle make these choices. Let's start the next chapter with all the good stuff . . .

A NOTE ON FASTING

Fasting! You mean starving yourself?! That's a bit of an extreme way to lose weight, don't you think? That's exactly what I thought the first time a friend told me about it. But then, like everything else related to nutrition and fitness, I figured I would do a bit of research on the concept and decide if it was something that I should test myself before disregarding it.

I researched fasting quite extensively, possibly because everything I read seemed so interesting. I then tested two different types of fasting: intermittent fasting, and full-day fasting. I will go into my experiences with these two methods, but first let's look at why you would even consider 'starving yourself' to improve your health.

Firstly, fasting is not just about losing weight (although you will lose body fat) — it has far more incredible health benefits. It is thought to decrease your risk of developing Type 2 diabetes, cardiovascular disease and dementia; it can lower your blood pressure and cholesterol levels; it can boost your immune system; and it is even thought to make you live longer! Essentially, fasting is a beneficial stressor, and when your body responds to this positive stress it becomes stronger and healthier.

In fact, the premise of fasting has some parallels with the paleo lifestyle. The cavemen and women we evolved from would have gone through periods of fasting all the time. Food wasn't so easy to come by — you couldn't just leave your cave and go down the road to the supermarket for some steak, veges and milk. In fact, being in a fully fed state all the time (which we generally are today) would have been extremely uncommon. Our bodies evolved to function best by being in fed states (after eating a meal) and then spending extended periods of time in fasted states (between meals).

So what happens to your body when you stop eating? For the first few hours, your body starts using all of the glycogen and fat that you have stored as energy. This is when all of that spare fat you have lining your body is used. You could argue that you haven't stopped eating, but you're just eating all of the food that your body has been storing.

After about twelve to eighteen hours it gets a bit more interesting. Your body starts to break down all the waste and damaged cells in your body and then it starts to repair itself.

Imagine it's the middle of winter, your house is freezing and you can't afford to have any sort of heating, so you decide to burn stuff that's lying around the house to keep warm. First you burn the crap that you don't really need. Well, your body does the same thing. First it burns the rubbish — the old cells, sick cells and decomposed tissue. It is the ultimate spring clean for your body! This process eliminates toxins and metabolic waste and at the same time turns them into heat and energy for the body.

While your body is getting rid of the old, sick and dead cells, it starts to repair itself. New, healthy cells are made and tissue is repaired. Your immune system gets a huge boost — white blood cells (the cells that fight sickness) are constantly battling against allergens and bacteria and often become damaged or sick themselves. It is when these cells become run down themselves that they aren't able to effectively fight off harmful things and you get sick. During fasting, white blood cells get a break from fighting and are able to heal themselves and be replaced by new ones, boosting your immune system and making you more resilient to illness.

The first technique I tried was intermittent fasting.

This is where you don't eat for between twelve and sixteen hours every day. The timing of this fasting window can be done any time of the day to fit in with your lifestyle. For me, I would fast between 8pm and midday the next day, and would then do a workout in my lunch-break on an empty stomach.

At first I found it a bit weird not eating breakfast — I'd had breakfast every day of my life! The first two or three days, I was watching the clock, waiting for 12pm to come round because I was so hungry (or thought I should be) but my body soon got used to the pattern. Eventually I found I didn't miss breakfast at all — I just wasn't really hungry in the mornings.

And, even though I had 'skipped' a meal, I found I had more energy throughout the day. I lost body fat while maintaining muscle mass, and I could exercise to the intensity level I wanted. I found that this worked well with my body and I felt great — I continued intermittent fasting most days for a few months and was probably the leanest I have ever been.

I don't consistently do intermittent fasting any more as I find that it doesn't fit in with my lifestyle. First thing in the morning is the only time I can find to exercise, and I like to eat soon after exercising. However, on days when I don't exercise in the morning, I do fast — I basically go without breakfast and make lunch my first meal of the day.

I then experimented with full-day fasting. The first time I tried it I actually failed — I started very ambitiously by trying to do a full two-day fast. And, being the hero that I thought I was, I decided to really test my body and continue to exercise twice a day just as I would normally do.

The first day was fine: I did a lunchtime and evening workout no problem. The second day I did my lunchtime workout and then about an hour later I began to feel very lightheaded. This freaked me out, as I thought I might pass out, so I figured it would be best to have some food and break my fast. It wouldn't have been a good look having the gym instructor, who was supposedly healthy, pass out because he had been starving himself!

I have since done many full-day fasts. I like to do one every week or two. I generally do them on days when I'm not exercising or am only doing moderate exercise. I also sometimes do full two-day fasts, which I find pretty easy now; I just make sure I'm not too active on those days. During these fasts I ingest nothing but water and sometimes herbal teas. Some people have different rules (for example, they might allow black coffee) but it's completely up to you. I choose to only have water as I know that I am not ingesting any substance that is going to have an effect on my body.

I do these fasts for the main purpose of boosting my immune system and cleaning up my body. We ingest a lot of toxins and bad stuff every day, which over time build up, damage cells, make you sick and basically disrupt your body from performing at its best. I like to think that, by fasting, I'm helping to get rid of all the bad stuff in my body, giving it a chance to recharge and repair — almost like a reset button, re-starting my body fresh and healthy.

I recommend doing a bit of further research on fasting as it's fascinating stuff. A really good short BBC documentary (for those of you who like to watch and learn) is called *Eat, Fast and Live Longer* by Dr Michael Mosley (find a link to watch this for free online at the back of the book).

In general I think both intermittent fasting and full-day fasting are both worth giving a crack. Intermittent fasting is a great way to lose body fat. Full fasting (for one or two days) is best for getting all of the metabolic and significant health benefits, along with losing body fat.

It's still considered a bit extreme, but I think fasting is going to become more and more prevalent in the next five or ten years; and I wouldn't be surprised if it becomes common to talk to friends who are fasting for their health. It makes sense to me, it's free, and it works. For me, less is definitely more.

Of course, if you have any concerns or existing medical conditions, it is important to talk about these with your doctor before giving fasting a nudge.

4. WHAT CAN I EAT?

So, now you know a bit more about the paleo lifestyle and its origins, you might be wanting to give it a try yourself. And you've probably got a lot of questions, like, 'Do I have to just eat heaps of meat? Do I have to give up cake? And can I eat as many fruits and veges as I want?'

Well, in short, the answers are: no, pretty much yes, and kind of. Let's look at what foods form the building blocks of the paleo lifestyle, and which ones you want to avoid if you want to get the most benefits. As I've said before, this is not a rule book, and I am not going to tell you, 'Yes, you have to eat a kilo of broccoli a day,' or, 'No, absolutely no milk in your coffee.' In the end, it's up to you what you do and don't eat, and how strict you want to be with your nutrition. But here are the basics.

When some people think 'paleo', they picture a bunch of cavemen tearing into a hunk of barbecued mammoth with not much in the way of veges on the side. In fact, while meat is a key nutrient source in the paleo lifestyle, being paleo doesn't give you a licence to eat as much meat as you can lay your hands on. Everything in moderation! But certainly meat, as in any balanced diet, is the main source of protein in the paleo lifestyle. Red meat like beef and lamb, poultry such as chicken and turkey, and fish of all kinds are all welcome on your paleo plate.

Where possible, and if you can afford it, the meat and poultry you eat should be organic and free range. And, with red meat, the best option is grass-fed. The great news for Kiwis is that virtually all the beef and lamb in our supermarkets and butcheries is grass-fed — unlike in the United States, for example, where cattle are reared on giant feedlots and fed corn and grains. So in New Zealand we're one step ahead already, without having to buy any fancy stuff.

Grass-fed meat not only tastes better and its production more humane, but it is far healthier for us compared to grain-fed meat. It is much higher in vitamins A and E, and contains far more omega-3 fatty acids and far fewer omega-6 fatty acids. It's this fatty-acid ratio that I see as the major benefit of grass-fed meat.

Both omega-3 and omega-6 fatty acids are essential

to maintain certain bodily functions and to aid in keeping you healthy, but they are required in different amounts. Omega-3 fatty acids help brain function, have an anti-inflammatory effect and can protect against heart disease. Omega-6 fatty acids, on the other hand, can actually have an inflammatory effect when there are too many of them in the body, and this can be a precursor to chronic diseases such as heart disease. In the past these chronic diseases have been linked to red-meat consumption in general, but now it seems the correlation is more to do with eating grain-fed beef. Just as we humans are not evolutionarily adapted to eat processed foods and sugars, cows are not adapted to eating processed grains as food — they are supposed to eat grass! So the healthiest beef and lamb comes from animals that have been allowed to roam around in lush paddocks, stare at you as you drive past them, and eat what nature intended them to.

The same goes for free-range poultry — or, even better, poultry with the SPCA Blue Tick, which certifies that animals have been farmed to the SPCA's high welfare standards. Healthy chickens that spend their lives roaming around eating natural foods are going to produce better-quality meat and eggs, without antibiotic and other chemical residues which negatively affect our bodies when we consume them.

The closer to nature the food you eat is, the better it is for you.

Likewise, fresh fish is the ideal, if you can find a good source that is affordable. Fresh-caught fish is the best if you happen to have your own gear and the time to get out on the water, but here in New Zealand the fish from the supermarket and fish shops is still pretty good. And even canned fish such as salmon is an OK option — just make sure it's from sustainable sources.

Seafood is OK too — shellfish like mussels, scallops and oysters, squid and prawns. Again, get it as fresh and local as you can.

One important thing to remember is that living a paleo lifestyle is not an excuse to go nuts and eat the Mad Butcher out of business. Paleo is not a high-protein diet; you don't need to eat any more meat than you would on a 'regular' eating regimen. Just because you are allowed to eat something doesn't mean you can go crazy on it. You need to get a range of nutrients from your food, and not overdose on protein.

And the other good news is the meat you eat doesn't have to be lean. You don't have to spend ages trimming the visible fat off your lamb chops before tossing them in the frying pan. Natural animal fats are good for us — our ancestors would have feasted on the fat of the animals they caught and killed, and would have gained vital nutrients from it. Our bodies need dietary fat for energy and cell growth, plus these fats help your body absorb some nutrients and produce important hormones.

Fat is a natural part of all animals and it's OK to eat it, despite what we might have been taught in the past about saturated fat. Plus, it's super tasty.

Speaking of tasty — bacon, even though it's a

TOO MUCH MEAT?

One common misperception of a paleo lifestyle is that you eat way too much meat. But, as I've said above, just because paleo incorporates meat doesn't mean that you have to eat a *lot* of meat. You can choose how much you want to eat: no one's forcing you to eat half a cow at every meal.

I do, however, believe that some people following this lifestyle possibly do eat more meat than they require and should probably eat more vegetables instead, especially green leafy ones.

One of the big arguments against not eating too much red meat is its sometimes suggested role in bowel-cancer rates. As with other nutritional studies, this comes down to which research you choose to believe.

I personally believe that eating meat doesn't cause bowel cancer, but rather that it is gluten that causes inflammation and slows down the function of the large intestine. This results in a very slow transit time for food through your digestive tract. This slow transit time means partially digested meat lingers in the large intestine and bowel and can damage the cells there.

Paleo is not about eating your weight in meat. It's about eating real food and avoiding foods that damage your body. Do some research, and make the decision that feels best for your body.

processed meat product, is most definitely still on the menu. I get mine from a butcher, who cures it himself. You need to be wary when buying bacon from supermarkets, as a lot of it has sugars, preservatives (nitrates are a common one) and water added to it. Check the label before buying it, or find a good butcher who makes a nice, naturally cured bacon. This will taste way better too.

VEGETABLES

Mother Nature has provided us with hundreds of vegetables of all different shapes, sizes and colours — green, red, yellow, orange, blue, purple and white. They all taste different and offer different health benefits, but the one thing that they have in common is that they are all good for us!

Green leafy vegetables such as cabbage, bok choy, broccoli, Brussels sprouts, silver beet and kale are the best vegetables for your body — these are the super-veges which many studies have suggested have anti-cancer properties and are so nutrient dense. Plus there are salad greens, like lettuce, mesclun and rocket, and all the other tasty vege delights, like courgettes and scallopini squash, cauliflower, carrots, capsicums, aubergines, asparagus … you'll never go hungry or unsatisfied as long as there are veges around.

They are all so good for you, in terms of their nutrient profiles, and each has specific health benefits. Here are a few veges that are super good for us.

→ **Kale:** It might not look like much, but kale is amazing. It's the richest vegetable source of vitamin K, and may help to reduce the risk of developing certain cancers. It's a fantastic source of calcium, chlorophyll, calcium, iron and vitamins A and C, too. Kale is low in calories and yet incredibly dense in nutrients. It's also a good source of minerals, copper, potassium, iron, manganese and phosphorus, as well as compounds which promote eye and skin health.

→ **Broccoli:** Known to benefit liver function and pro-mote natural detoxification. It is high in vitamin E and contains an excellent amount of vitamin C, which helps heal cuts and injuries and keep teeth and gums healthy. Broccoli also contains pantothenic acid (vitamin B5) and vitamin A, which work together to improve rough skin. Broccoli is also a good source of iron and other B vitamins and some studies have shown it to have anti-cancer properties.

→ **Spinach**: Popeye's favourite vegetable is an excellent source of vitamins A, C and E. It's also a good source of calcium, iron, potassium and protein, and contains choline, which supports healthy mental function.

→ **Asparagus:** Eat this if you want to age well. It has been shown to potentially prevent cognitive decline and is packed with antioxidants, which neutralise cell-damaging free radicals — another reason why it's a great anti-aging food. A very good source of fibre and vitamins A, C, E and K, asparagus also contains chromium, a trace mineral that assists insulin to transport glucose from the bloodstream into cells.

I love my veges and love coming up with new ways to eat them — have a look at the recipe section on pages 178–221 for some creative ways to make vegetables more exciting.

BAD VEGES

Because a paleo lifestyle avoids grains, vegetables can be used as substitutes for staples such as rice, bread and potatoes. 'But potatoes are a vegetable,' I hear you say. Well . . . kind of. Potatoes are a tuber, which is essentially a swollen plant root. They contain a lot of starch, and have a high GI (glycaemic index — see page 79), so are generally avoided as part of the paleo lifestyle. Remember — paleo isn't just about eating certain food groups but more about eating foods that are good for us and avoiding foods that aren't as good for us. We are lucky enough in New Zealand to have our very own low-GI sweet potato, the kumara, which is a great addition to many meals!

The other vegetables which are a bit of a no-no are beans (green beans as well as pulses like kidney beans, lentils and chickpeas) and peas. I know, I know, they're veges too, but in fact they are actually legumes, which means you are eating the seed of the plant. You see, plants can be tricky little customers, and they are a lot more biologically sophisticated than we give them credit for. Just like every other living thing, plants have a goal of living for as long as possible and procreating. Most living things have therefore developed defence mechanisms to help them do this — for example, skunks produce an unbearable scent spray to ward off predators, and we humans have the ability to fight off predators or run away. Plants obviously can't run away like animals, so they have developed other ways to protect themselves.

Legumes, peas and beans have developed the ability to make their predators (humans or other animals) sick. Their cells contain lectins, phytic acid and saponins. Lectins cause inflammation in the cells that make up the gut wall, and can lead to leaky gut, a terrible autoimmune disorder. Phytic acid prevents nutrients being absorbed in the gut — you can eat all the nutrients you want, but phytic acid will just cause them to pass right through you. Saponins are pretty nasty too — they also attack the cells of the gut wall and can help cause leaky gut. Once this happens, saponins, bacteria and other toxins start leaking into your bloodstream. An immediate effect is that saponins start destroying the cell membranes of your red blood cells (as well as leading to general inflammation in your body). After that, all sorts of other bad things start happening. No thanks.

VEGES AS SUBSTITUTES

The good news about most veges is that they can be used to create substitutes for foods which you might have decided not to eat, such as pasta and rice.

Courgettes make a great pasta substitute — courgetti (courgette spaghetti), anyone? — and you can slice carrots into long, thin strips to cover with a nice meat sauce, too.

Broccoli and cauliflower can be broken up into little pieces and cooked to make vegetable 'rice' or 'couscous' (see page 212 for my Cauliflower Couscous recipe), for times when you are missing that added texture that traditional carbs bring to a meal.

If you, like me, were brought up thinking that you need all of these carbs from pasta, rice and bread for energy, then think again. Vegetables contain valuable carbohydrates too — but in a far more nutritious, digestible and bio-accessible form than processed or starchy carbs. (For more information about exercise and nutrition, see chapter 10.)

FRUIT

Fruit gets the big tick too, but with one proviso: you can't run around eating loads of it all day. Fruit still contains sugar — although in its natural form, fructose — and too much of it is not a good thing, as you can easily consume more energy than you need. (Plus, you know what happens when you eat too many kiwifruit . . .) Sure, our ancestors ate fruit — they probably loved the sweetness as much as we do, although before the rise of agriculture naturally occurring fruits wouldn't have been anywhere near as big, sweet and juicy as the varieties we know today are, which have been altered through selective breeding — but, importantly, fruit was both hard to find and highly seasonal. There was no going down to the fruit shop and buying grapes from Mexico, apricots from Turkey and oranges from California during the Paleolithic period.

When living a paleo lifestyle, it's important to respect seasonality and eat those fruits which are naturally available in your area at that time of the year. Sure, it means winter is a bit lean compared to the abundance of summer, but there's still pears, kiwifruit, mandarins . . . The one big exception to seasonality, which I personally would find difficult to give up, is bananas. They are a great source of low-GI energy and the perfect snack. If you are exercising regularly, bananas are a superfood. They are high in potassium and magnesium, making them a great electrolyte replenisher — I like to think of bananas as a natural-food version of a sports drink.

Just try to keep your fruit intake to two pieces a day — unless you are working out, in which case you can probably slip in another banana. And, remember, fruit juice and dried fruit are cheating. You wouldn't sit down and eat five oranges at one time, so don't drink them in a glass. Even 'natural' sugar can be bad for you if you consume more of it than your body needs for its energy output.

EGGS

I love eggs. They are so versatile, tasty and they are one of the most amazing foods from a nutritional point of view. They contain all nine essential amino acids — the building blocks of the proteins our body needs to survive and thrive — and are very high in protein. I like to think of eggs as containing everything nature needs to grow. After all, that's how a baby chicken is made. The fertilised egg is laid and in the space of three weeks a tiny little embryo grows into a fully developed chick, having only used the yolk and albumen (egg white) as fuel to grow. So all that nutritional goodness that goes into making a new life — which doesn't of course happen in the unfertilised chicken eggs that we eat — can go into your body.

Eggs got a bad rap a few years ago, with some studies suggesting that the fats the yolks contain increased human cholesterol levels, and a lot of people got scared off eating them. However, a lot of that research has been superseded as our knowledge of cholesterol has become more sophisticated, and eggs are definitely back on the menu. If you have a family history of cholesterol problems or existing high cholesterol levels then perhaps you may want to keep an eye on your egg intake, but I don't think it's essential. I personally have up to five eggs a day a couple of times a week.

NUTS AND SEEDS

Back in hunter-gatherer days, edible nuts and seeds would have formed an important part of our ancestors' diets. They were a nutrient- and energy-dense food source which would have provided an important boost in terms of good fats and vitamins. Yes, nuts are high in fat, but it's good fat: heart-healthy unsaturated fats and omega-3 fatty acids which help to lower cholesterol and regulate heart rhythms. They also contain vitamin E, and may contain plant sterols, which are also believed to lower cholesterol. Walnuts, almonds, macadamia nuts, Brazil nuts, hazelnuts, cashews — they're all good, nutritious, energy-dense snacks that are handy for on-the-go consumption.

But don't go too nuts — just like meat, the fact that most nuts and seeds were available to our ancestors is not enough in itself to justify overconsumption. They are quite energy-dense, and you don't want to be consuming more energy than your body requires — otherwise the excess energy can be stored in your body as fat. And, even though nuts have a lot of good nutrients, some also have small amounts of anti-nutrients like phytic acid and omega-6 fatty acids, which are fine in small doses but could cause problems to some if consumed in excess.

Seeds are great too: think pumpkin seeds, sunflower seeds, flaxseed. Most contain healthy minerals such as zinc and magnesium along with omega-3 fatty acids.

Both nuts and seeds are great for adding flavour and texture to meals, especially for sparking up salads. They are also good for snacks — in small quantities, as it's easy to consume more energy than you need without realising it when you're nibbling on something so small and tasty.

HEALTHY OILS

Because fat is not the enemy in a paleo lifestyle, you're free to use healthy oils in your cooking. The more pure, unprocessed and natural the oil the better. Highly processed vegetable oils, such as canola, sunflower and soybean oil, are made using an industrial process which involves the oil being stripped out of the vegetable product using a solvent like hexane, then washed with chemical soap and bleached. Still want to fry your dinner in it?

Natural oils like olive and coconut oil, which are

just squeezed out of the flesh of the plant, are a much healthier alternative.

Coconut oil is really great to cook with — it has a very high smoke point so it doesn't burn very easily. I alternate between using it and olive oil — coconut oil does have a slightly, well, coconutty taste which doesn't suit all foods. Coconut oil also has a melting point of around 20 degrees Celsius, so in New Zealand it's a solid for much of the year, and olive oil can be more convenient to use in some instances.

Although a strict paleo regime excludes dairy products, I am a bit of a sucker for butter, and use it from time to time when cooking. It just tastes so good! We are so lucky in New Zealand to have access to butter which is so natural and produced from grass-fed cows' milk. We also produce some amazing organic olive oil and other nut oils which are super good. It's great to be able to use products which have been produced just down the road, rather than in some big factory overseas.

So there, look at all those great, wholesome foods that are compatible with a paleo lifestyle! But you might have noticed that a few things which are central to your current diet are missing. Read on, and let's find out why starchy carbs, grains, refined sugars and processed foods are on the way out of your life.

5. WHAT FOODS
SHOULD I AVOID?

If you're the person always reaching for the bread, or serving yourself big helpings of rice or pasta, then I'm afraid I've got bad news for you: you're going to be looking for some substitutes. But the good news is that these foods aren't excluded just because I'm feeling mean — it's because they actually harm our bodies and have negative effects on our overall health and wellbeing. So I'm actually doing you a massive favour. And, from experience, I can tell you that, once you've said *sayonara* to grains and starchy carbs, it won't be long before you wonder why you ever ate them in the first place.

So, what foods should you avoid if you're wanting to follow a paleo lifestyle?

CEREAL GRAINS

This is the biggie. Basically this covers all grains and their by-products — basically anything made with flour. So that means no bread, no pasta, no couscous.

Put quite simply, before the widespread adoption of agriculture about 10,000 years ago, human beings didn't eat cereal grains. Now we hoover them down like there's no tomorrow. They're cheap, they're abundant and we've grown used to the taste and texture, especially in a bread-heavy Western diet. And they're often the hardest thing for people to give up when they are adopting a paleo lifestyle, because of their very ubiquity. A lot of people can't imagine a day without cereal for breakfast, a sandwich for lunch and bread or pasta with dinner.

SO WHY ARE GRAINS SO BAD FOR US?

Three main reasons, really: phytates, lectins and gluten.

→ Phytates: These compounds, also found in lesser quantities in nuts and seeds, are not inherently damaging, but they do bind to dietary minerals and prevent them from being absorbed. They're not as harmful as gluten or lectins if the rest of your diet is mineral rich. (Tip: to help break down phytates, you can soak food in yoghurt, buttermilk or water combined with lemon juice or vinegar.)

→ Lectins: These are so small and hard to digest that they tend to bioaccumulate (become concentrated) inside your body. They damage the gut lining,

73

WHEAT
A quick history lesson

- - - - - - - - - - -

C. 10,000 YEARS AGO	Wheat first used as food
C. 8500 YEARS AGO	Man begins to cultivate wheat
C. 5000 YEARS AGO	Egyptians the first to make bread
C. 2000 YEARS AGO	Bread a staple of the Roman diet
C. 1200	Windmills used for grinding wheat to flour
1400-1600	Bread production and consumption grows during the Middle Ages
1760-1830	The Industrial Revolution – cheap food is needed for the masses and bread becomes a staple
1850-1900	Flour refined to make bread last longer. New technology makes bread easier and cheaper to produce
1900s	Crop breeding and science increase wheat production
1930s-1940s	Wheat touted as a healthy option during food shortages
1951-1990	World wheat production increases dramatically due to productivity improvements worldwide (from 1 tonne per hectare in 1951 to 2.5 tonnes per hectare by 1995). Consumption rises accordingly
TODAY	Wheat is one of the most cultivated crops in the world

which leads to leaky gut and other disorders (see page 98 for more on gut health). Lectins also cause leptin resistance, which means that your hunger signal is suppressed, so you feel hungry even when your body has had more than enough calories. Lectins are resistant to heat and digestive enzymes and can bind to almost all cell types, causing damage to tissues and organs.

→ Gluten: This is the big one. It's talked about so much — there are gluten-free diets, books, events and sections in supermarkets. But what exactly is gluten and why should we avoid it?

GLUTEN

Gluten is a complex protein found in wheat (which was first domesticated in the Middle East around 12,000 years ago) and other grains including barley, rye and oats. In bread-making, gluten is basically the glue that gives the bread dough its elasticity. When the yeast ferments and produces carbon dioxide, it's gluten that holds the whole lot together and creates the end product: a baked loaf, with that familiar lightness and texture. Modern technology and breeding have increased the amount of gluten present in farmed wheat, so that wheat now contains about 80 per cent gluten.

Gluten is a lectin, which is a protein compound produced by plants to make their seeds hard to digest — a bit like the saponins produced by legumes. Lectins damage the lining of the gut, making it hard to absorb nutrients and leading to gut leakage, which is as disgusting as it sounds. The gut reacts to protect itself and this causes inflammation, which can be experienced as discomfort, but more likely rumbles away unnoticed, potentially contributing to chronic autoimmune diseases such as cancers and multiple sclerosis.

That's not to say that most people are what we'd call 'gluten intolerant' and are going to have a major reaction and get really sick from eating gluten. Gluten affects all of us differently. Some people may experience no noticeable problems, whereas others may experience negative effects — things such as bloating and diarrhoea, feeling tired and even moodiness and depression. The most serious form of gluten intolerance is called coeliac disease, an autoimmune disease, where the body's immune system starts attacking normal tissue, causing a plethora of serious problems.

A lot of research is coming out which shows that, even if you don't physically feel that something is wrong in your gut, you will actually be doing your brain a massive favour by putting down that sandwich. This notion that grains and gluten are harmful for your brain is gaining momentum, with some scientists now believing that diets high in grains (especially modern wheat) may be one of the causes of Alzheimer's disease, dementia, migraines and ADHD.

The three big gluten-containing grains are wheat, rye and barley. Oats don't contain the same levels of gluten (and you can get gluten-free varieties) but people who are strictly paleo avoid them as well, as part of cutting out all grains.

GRAIN BRAIN

⟋⟍⟋⟍

I really enjoyed reading a book called *Grain Brain* (2013) by Dr David Perlmutter. It looks at multiple ongoing studies that link high-sugar, high-glycaemic diets full of grains and gluten to the insulin dysfunction in the brain that causes cognitive impairment and Alzheimer's disease.

I recommend this book very highly for anyone who is interested in the health of their brain. However, for those who can't be bothered reading it, I will sum it up quite simply by saying this: if you want your brain to be functioning at its best when you're 80 then don't eat grains — or at least eat far less — from now on. Easy.

RICE

'What about rice?' you might ask. 'That's gluten free. Why can't I eat that?' Yep, good question, and there's not a straightforward answer.

Some people who follow a paleo lifestyle avoid rice altogether, because it is a farmed grain which wasn't available to our ancestors. But white rice can be considered a 'safe starch'. Each grain of rice in its natural state — what we think of as brown rice — has a protective coating round the outside of each kernel that is basically pure starch. It is this outer coating which contains all the nasties that can irritate your gut, while

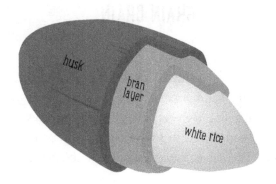

the white-rice kernel inside can be a useful carbohydrate which doesn't provide stress on the body's digestive system, especially if you are exercising a lot and need some extra carbs.

However, because white rice is made up entirely of starchy sugars, it contains virtually no micronutrients — vitamins, minerals, anything. All it is is a source of fuel, but not of any goodness.

The other good reason to avoid starchy, grain-based carbs like bread and rice is that they often have a high GI (see opposite page), which means they can be converted by the body into blood sugar quickly and easily. This causes blood-sugar spikes and dips, and corresponding surges of insulin — the body's way of breaking down sugars in the blood.

If your body gets into the habit of producing insulin to deal with excess blood sugar, it can reach a state of insulin resistance — where the body's cells

WHAT'S THIS GI THING?

GI stands for 'glycemic index', which basically means a measure of how much the carbohydrates in foods raise blood glucose (or sugar) levels. The GI was originally developed to help people with diabetes manage their condition, but researchers found it could be useful for the general population too, to give them an idea of the effects of different foods on their blood glucose levels, and therefore on their overall health and wellbeing. Basically, the lower the GI, the more slowly a carbohydrate is broken down during digestion and releases its sugars into the bloodstream. Low-GI foods release glucose at a slow and steady rate, helping to avoid blood sugar spikes and dips.

Eating paleo cuts out a lot of high-GI carbohydrates like white rice and potatoes. Most carbohydrates in a paleo lifestyle are sourced from low-GI foods such as vegetables and fruit. However, there are some low-GI foods which are not paleo, such as wholegrain bread and pasta, so stick to the paleo rules first before following GI ratings.

Scientists have tested hundreds of foods, and you can find lists of GI ratings online or download an app to help you check out what you're eating and make good decisions.

stop responding to insulin and doing what they are supposed to do — and eventually you will develop Type 2 diabetes.

As we are all aware, Type 2 diabetes is a serious and growing health problem in our society — nearly a quarter of a million Kiwis suffer from it — and it's purely to do with diet. We are doing it to ourselves. So do yourself a favour and turn your back on starchy carbs — your body will thank you for it.

I personally don't eat rice, but I believe it's probably OK to eat in small quantities, if that's what you want to do. The traditional diets of many Asian cultures, such as the Japanese, include small quantities of rice without causing serious health problems. But here's the key: they aren't wolfing down massive bowls of it. We Westerners tend to serve ourselves huge quantities of rice even with healthy vegetable stir-fries. Think how much rice is in a piece of sushi, or in the little compartment of a bento box, and cut down your portions.

REFINED SUGAR

This is the other biggie. As with starchy carbohydrates and cereal grains, refined sugar plays havoc with your blood-sugar levels, leading to insulin resistance and Type 2 diabetes. After eating it you get a big peak, but an even bigger dip, which leaves you feeling sleepy and reaching for even more sugar — it's a vicious circle.

Sugar is the big bogey-man in the media at the

moment, with movies like *That Sugar Film* and books like *Sweet Poison* by David Gillespie and *Pure, White and Deadly* by John Yudkin hitting the headlines and the bestseller lists. And for good reason: if you haven't yet watched *That Sugar Film* I seriously urge you to — it's eye-opening in an entertaining way. More and more research is emerging, showing how bad refined sugar is for the body, and the damage we have been doing to ourselves with our addiction to sweet things.

We have had the 'fat is making us fat' message shoved down our throats for so many years, but finally we are beginning to understand that fat is not the enemy that it was thought to be; really, it is sugar that is making us sick, overweight and, essentially, killing us. Sugar has a massive part to play in increasing rates of obesity and heart disease — the single biggest killer in New Zealand, accounting for more than 30 per cent of deaths annually. Every 90 minutes, a Kiwi dies from heart disease.

Now, do you really want to drink that Coke? Put it down and step away slowly . . .

We all like a bit of sweetness in our lives. When living a paleo lifestyle you can get that from naturally occurring sugars such as those found in dates, maple syrup and honey.

Artificial sweeteners are, of course, off-limits. There's no point in just cutting something out of your diet and replacing it with chemicals — sure, artificial sweeteners have few or no calories, but paleo is not about calorie-counting. It's about eating foods that we were designed to eat and avoiding foods that harm us. Every now and then our ancestors would have found some honey (and probably got well stung in the process of procuring it). If they lived in certain parts of the world they would sometimes have eaten dates. But you can be certain that they weren't sitting around eating sugary muesli bars, soft drinks, cakes, lollies, bakery goods, ice cream . . .

I'm not saying don't eat these things ever again. I'm just saying think about it, with the knowledge that these things are seriously harming your body. And don't think that 'diet' versions of these things are OK — I would argue that often the diet versions are even *worse*! How many chemicals made in a laboratory do you think it takes to make diet soft drinks as sweet as the full-sugar ones?

So, what can you eat if you just have to have sweetness? You can substitute refined sugar in your cooking with unprocessed natural sugars such as honey or maple syrup (make sure it's the real stuff, not just maple-flavoured syrup), or add sweetness to baking with fresh dates and fruit. But the biggest question to ask yourself is, 'Do I need to be eating sweet stuff all the time?'

Having a sweet tooth is really just a habit. It's actually ridiculous when you think about it: having a 'sweet tooth' is not a thing! We say it like it's some sort of excuse or explanation for why we like sweet, sugary foods. 'Yeah, I ate that whole block of chocolate because I have a sweet tooth' — as if it is some sort of personal trait that some people are born with and others aren't. It's not!

Part of adopting a paleo lifestyle is rethinking that dependence on the sweet stuff and getting pleasure and satisfaction from other foods, rather than just downing some sugar to get a hit. After a while you won't even crave sugar and sweet things like you used to.

I know it's hard when you're surrounded by it, especially if your friends, flatmates or family haven't made the decision to eat more healthily. I'm not immune to temptation either — if my flatmates bring home a bag of those mini Toblerones and they are sitting on the coffee table while we're watching TV . . . well, I'm only human. I'm probably going to have one! The key is to keep temptation to a minimum by not having sugary food around you or in the house. You're less likely to stuff chocolate in your face if you have to go out to the gas station to get some.

Another thing you really need to look out for is all of the 'hidden' sugar that lives in many of the 'healthy' packaged and processed foods on our supermarket shelves. Here's a quick example that I'm going to borrow from *That Sugar Film*: one 'healthy' breakfast consisting of a bowl of cereal topped with low-fat yoghurt and a glass of apple juice can contain more than 20 teaspoons of sugar! That's crazy! And that is just one example of how we have been led to believe that some foods are healthy or nutritious for us when really they are just packaged poison for our bodies.

Have a read of some of those food labels next time you're walking down the breakfast aisle or in the muesli bar section of the supermarket, and what you find will quite possibly surprise and disgust you. (For more on food labelling, see page 86.) Sucrose, maltose, dextrose, maltodextrin, malt syrup, molasses, corn syrup . . . they're all just ways of saying sugar. Which leads me on to . . .

PROCESSED FOODS

This is where things get really scary. Processed foods tend to come in shiny, colourful bags, boxes or jars. They are 'foods' — and I use inverted commas deliberately — that have generally been engineered to taste as good as possible, last as long as possible, and be as addictive as possible, all while costing the least possible amount of money to produce. This 'food' is not grown but rather created in laboratories, by workers wearing safety goggles and white lab coats, holding a smoking beaker in one hand and a clipboard in the other (probably).

In addition to going through many complex production steps to get them to taste 'good' and last a long time, processed foods often contain additives, artificial flavourings and other chemical ingredients that your body will be better off without.

You can determine just how processed foods are by looking at their ingredients lists. I'll go into more detail on this in the food labels section on page 86, but the general rules are:

→ The longer the ingredients list, the more processed a food is likely to be.

→ The more words you don't recognise, the more processed a food is likely to be.
→ The more numbers there are, the more processed a food is likely to be.

Here is an example of the ingredients of a widely popular breakfast cereal marketed to children all over the world.

INGREDIENTS: Sugar, cornflour blend (wholegrain yellow cornflour, degerminated yellow cornflour), wheat flour, wholegrain oat flour, oat fibre, soluble corn fibre, contains 2 per cent or less of partially hydrogenated vegetable oil (coconut, soybean and/or cottonseed), salt, red 40, natural flavour, blue 2, turmeric colour, yellow 6, annatto colour, blue 1, BHT for freshness. Vitamins and minerals: Vitamin C (sodium ascorbate and ascorbic acid), niacinamide, reduced iron, zinc oxide, vitamin B6 (pyridoxine hydrochloride), vitamin B2 (riboflavin), vitamin B1 (thiamin hydrochloride), vitamin A palmitate, folic acid, vitamin D, vitamin B12

You can see why this stuff is scary! Millions of children are ingesting these chemicals — not to mention a truckload of sugar, which is the primary ingredient — every single day and it may be many years before we find out the long-term effects of doing so. Personally, I don't want to wait and find out first-hand so I just don't put that shit in my body — and I feel way better for it.

By avoiding processed foods you will also reduce your salt intake. Salt (and sugar) is frequently added to processed foods to make them taste better, and is often talked about as something we should restrict in our diet because of its association with high blood pressure. But you don't need to worry too much about your salt intake if you have cut out processed foods and are eating a wide range of natural wholefoods, as you will generally be consuming very little added salt.

TIP: Processed foods are usually found in the central aisles of the supermarket. Try to do most of your shopping around the outside walls — in the fresh fruit and vegetable and meat sections, without being sucked into the vortex of crap in the middle. Better still, find a good local butcher and greengrocer and give them your patronage.

READING LABELS

The aim of a paleo lifestyle is to eat foods which are as natural as possible, so you shouldn't be eating too much packaged stuff. But I know life isn't always that simple, and from time to time you are going to find yourself eating packaged foods that have been made in a factory rather than grown on a tree or raised on a farm. So be aware of what is in the products you might find on your supermarket shelves.

The trouble with processed foods is that they have usually had chemicals added to them to increase their shelf life or to improve their colour, texture or taste. And when I say chemicals, I'm basically saying artificial, non-food ingredients. Look at the label, and

WHAT ARE MACRONUTRIENTS?

Nutrients are substances found in foods, which the body uses for energy, growth and maintaining basic bodily functions. Those that are needed in the body in large amounts are called macronutrients, and there are three which the human body requires: carbohydrates (sugars), lipids (fats) and proteins.

Each of these macronutrients provides a different amount of energy to the body: carbohydrates and proteins produce around 17 kilojoules per gram, and lipids 38 kilojoules per gram.

As you will have worked out by now (hopefully!), if you're following a paleo lifestyle you want to choose foods which are high in protein and good fats but low in carbs and sugar. (See more on reading nutritional labels on page 89.)

anything that's identified by a number (e.g. 951, which is the artificial sweetener aspartame, or 210, which is a preservative) is a chemical. And you don't want to be eating that stuff. Our bodies aren't meant to ingest it and it can only have negative effects on us.

If you're going to adopt a paleo lifestyle, you're probably going to become one of those food nerds who reads food-ingredient labels pretty carefully. Sorry, but that comes with the territory! But once you know what you're looking at it is actually quite interesting, and kind of makes you look smarter. And, trust me, you're going to be shocked once you start looking at what's really in some of the foods you have been eating for years!

So, what do you look for when you look at a food label or nutrition panel? For me, because I am not trying to lose weight, paleo is not about calorie counting. What I am really interested in is what's in a certain food — whether or not the ingredients are good or bad for my body — and also its macronutrient profile, which means how much protein, carbohydrate (and therefore sugars) and fat it contains, and in what ratios.

If it's clearly paleo, then I know I can eat it, and I don't worry too much about the macronutrient profile. But if one or two ingredients aren't paleo then I need to have a good look at the nutrition it's providing so I can make a choice about whether or not I want to put it into my body.

Generally, I'm looking for foods which are high in protein and fat but low in carbs and sugar. For example, if I was going to eat some non-paleo chocolate, I would look for one containing lots of cocoa butter and cocoa solids, and the lowest amount of added sugar — something like an 80 per cent dark chocolate.

It can be hard work and quite time-consuming at first, but you'll soon get to know which products fit in with how you want to eat and are going to give you the best nutritional value.

NUTRITIONAL LABEL BREAKDOWN

In New Zealand, the panel must contain information about seven key components: energy, protein, fat, saturated fat, carbohydrates, sugars and sodium.

NUTRITIONAL INFORMATION
Servings per packet: 1
Serving size: 125 g

Average Quantity	Per Serving	Per 100 g
Energy	859.6 kj	687.7 kj
Protein	6.8 g	5.4 g
Fat – total	10.8 g	8.6 g
– saturated	6.7 g	5.4 g
– trans	0 g	0 g
Carbohydrate - total	21.6 g	17.3 g
– sugars	20.2 g	16.2 g
Sodium	77.3 mg	61.8 mg
Calcium	185.3 mg	148.2 mg

You can use the quantities in the per 100 g column to compare with other, similar products.

Ingredients
Skim milk concentrate, Sugar, Cocoa solids (7%), Cream, Chilli powder, Cultures (including *L. Acidophilus* & *bifidus*), **Thickener (1442)**, Flavour, **Preservative (200)**.

Ingredients are always listed in descending order of quantity, so the fact that sugar is second on this list means the product is really high in it — 20.2 g per serving works out to be 4 teaspoons!

The number of the food additive should always be listed after the name. Check online to find out what they are — or just put the box back on the shelf and find something that has no numbers.

Usually if a flavour is natural it will say so on the label, as this is a selling point. So, chances are, this one is not . . .

HOW THE INGREDIENTS BIT WORKS

All of the ingredients in a product have to be listed on the packaging, in descending order of quantity. Sometimes the key ingredients are listed with a percentage, indicating how much of that ingredient is actually in the product.

Fat, sugar and salt may be identified in ingredients lists under other names. Beware when shopping!

→ *Fat* may be listed as: animal oil or fat, vegetable oil or fat, butter fat, shortening, milk solids, Copha, chocolate, tallow, lard.

→ *Sugar* may be listed as: sucrose, glucose, fructose, lactose, maltose, dextrose, golden syrup, corn syrup, honey, malt, molasses.

→ *Salt* may be listed as: rock salt, vegetable salt, baking soda, baking powder, sodium, sodium bicarbonate, monosodium glutamate (MSG), stock cubes, yeast extract.

➤ TIP: A level teaspoon of sugar weighs 4 grams. Watch out for labels that say 'No added sugar' — all it means is that the manufacturers didn't add any, but don't assume that means the product contains *no* sugar. It could still contain lots of natural sugar, such as in dried fruit, honey or fruit juices. Check the nutritional information panel for the actual amount of sugar it contains.

A NOTE ABOUT STEVIA

There is a lot of chat on the internet about the sweetener Stevia and whether or not it can be included in a paleo diet. Some articles say it's OK, since it comes naturally from a plant and our ancestors could have chewed the leaves to enjoy the sweet taste. Some say it's not OK — the way we purchase Stevia today, it's highly processed, usually in a powder form and is a long way from its natural state.

Our bodies are not designed or evolved to handle calorie-free sweeteners — be they natural or artificial. Experiencing a sweet taste from a food that is not going to provide glucose confounds our body's sugar-handling process. Australian nutritionist Kate Skinner, author of the health blog Nutrition By Nature (nutritionbynature.com.au), explains how eating a sugar-free sweetener like Stevia can trick the body into a state of hypoglycaemia:

> Stevia is 'sweet' on the palate, so the body assumes it is receiving sugar and primes itself to do so. Glucose is cleared from the bloodstream and blood sugars drop, but no real sugar/glucose is provided to the body to compensate. When this happens, adrenaline and cortisol surge to mobilize sugar from other sources (liver and muscle glycogen, or protein, or body tissue) to bring blood glucose back up.

Stevia isn't going to have this exteme effect on everyone, but the frequent release of stress hormones like adrenalin and cortisol is damaging to our overall health. We have enough stress in our busy lives without encouraging our bodies to produce extra stress hormones!

But I guess I am a bit biased — the main reason I don't like Stevia is that I don't like the taste.

Unless you're going to plant your own stevia orchard in the back garden, harvest and produce your own sweetener, it's not really a very 'natural' product. That being said, it is still far better for you than any chemical artificial sweetener.

A much better thing to do is to train yourself to enjoy the flavour of tea or coffee without sweetener, and use honey or maple syrup in baking. Try to stay away from foods which rely on something being added to give them sweetness. Replacing processed sugar with sweetener, whether it's from a 'natural' source or not, is just continuing to feed your addiction to sweetness. Knock it on the head.

KICKING THE SUGAR HABIT

It doesn't matter if it's natural or artificial — when you eat something sweet, it lights up the same areas of your brain, as if you've taken a drug. And probably the very first time you ate something sweet — long, long before you can even remember — your brain filed that experience away as, 'Oooh! Yes please!' and it's been searching for that hit ever since.

The good news is you can retrain your brain to not crave sweet stuff, just by eating less and less of it.

You might be sitting there thinking, 'Oh, that's easy for him to say.' But, trust me, I know what it's like to give up sugar. I've always been a real sucker for chocolate — I mean, who isn't? So when I decided to follow a paleo lifestyle I thought that I would really struggle to give up chocolate, and initially I did. But after about three weeks I noticed that after dinner I began to just simply not feel like I 'needed' something sweet to complete the day.

I think it is part chemical addiction and part habit. Either way, you just have to have faith that once you break the craving cycle you simply will not crave sweetness like you used to. It is actually that easy. (You'll be pleased to know that the team at CleanPaleo is working on creating a paleo chocolate made from raw cacao and coconut sugar. You'd want to keep it for treats rather than eating it every day, but it tastes damn good!)

It's also really important to understand that sugar hides in drinks. It's actually very scary when you realise how much sugar is in some 'everyday' drinks. Have a look at the diagram over the page to get an idea.

When I was at high school in Christchurch, I got into the habit of having a can of Coke every night with my dinner. (Looking back, I can't believe my mum let me do that!) I didn't really think about what it was doing to me — you don't when you're that age — until one day I went to the dentist. He had a look in my mouth, shook his head and asked if I ate lots of lollies. 'No,' I said proudly. And did I brush my teeth twice a day? 'Yes.' Hmmm. So that left one thing . . . did I drink much Coke? 'Um, yes.' Turns out it wasn't just the sugar in the Coke that was damaging my teeth; it was also the acid in it, which was eating away the enamel. Coke has a pH or acid level of around 2.5; by comparison, battery acid has a pH of 1, and pure water is neutral, with a pH of 7.

Needless to say, that scared me off drinking Coke, and now my teeth are in really good condition. Interestingly, though, it was the tooth thing that did it for me — I wasn't worried about the other effects the Coke might be having on my body because that was before I learnt about all this stuff. But, looking back, I'm so glad I kicked that habit early on, as I can only imagine what havoc all of that sugar would have been playing on my body, brain, hormones and sleep.

DAIRY PRODUCTS

Dairy, much like grains, is another food group forming a cornerstone of our Western diet — and also of the New Zealand economy — that is coming under increasing pressure from scientific research into nutrition.

The main energy source in dairy is lactose, which is a sugar — a 'natural' one, sure, but one that our bodies find hard to digest. Different studies suggest up to three-quarters of adults have difficulty digesting lactose, due to an insufficiency of the enzyme lactase in their

HOW MUCH SUGAR REALLY IS IN THOSE DRINKS?

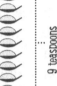
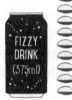

FIZZY DRINK (375ml)

9 teaspoons

ENERGY DRINK (250ml)

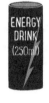

6 teaspoons

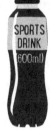
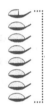

SPORTS DRINK (600ml)

7 ½ teaspoons

FRUIT JUICE (200ml)

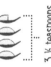

3 ½ teaspoons

COCONUT WATER (250ml)

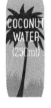

2 ½ teaspoons

digestive systems — it's especially common in Eastern cultures, where people aren't brought up drinking a lot of milk.

While some people suffer quite major symptoms of lactose intolerance — farting, tummy pain, bloating, diarrhoea — many people have only minor symptoms, but their guts are struggling nonetheless. It seems that people produce different amounts of lactase, so some people can drink as much milk as they like and experience no adverse effects, while others will have a bit of a 'funny tummy' after having milk on their cereal or a latte at morning tea (see more about coffees on page 150).

Babies and young children produce more lactase and are able to tolerate dairy products more easily than adults, but that's because they need to be able to digest human breast milk — not cow breast milk. Human breast milk has a very different nutritional composition to cow's milk: it's much lower in protein, higher in fat, much higher in carbohydrate and has heaps less calcium.

When you think about it, drinking cow's milk — which many of us do every day — is a bit weird. After all, it is a food which mummy cows make to feed their babies. Baby cows, that is. So why are *we* drinking it? And I know this also sounds quite weird, but it makes me wonder, 'Would it actually make more sense for us to drink human breast milk?' When most people think about that they are completely grossed out, but I just can't help but feel, all ethical aspects aside, that it would be more natural for a species to consume the milk from its own species. (Just to be clear though, I'm not suggesting there be milking sheds for humans!)

For all these reasons, and because farming animals for milk is the result of a post-agricultural society, dairy products should be avoided or minimised when living a paleo lifestyle. If you're going to be strict about it, you should avoid all forms of dairy, but I make a few exceptions: I sometimes have cream in my coffee, at times I cook with butter, and I do eat cheese. Because these things taste good, and I like them, and I don't feel any adverse effects from them. I believe in moderation, and in not denying myself. But you can make your own choices, and cut out what you feel you can.

BEANS, PEAS, PEANUTS AND OTHER LEGUMES

As discussed already, the saponins in these foods can cause damage to your gut. There are plenty of other good vege and nut options which are just fine to eat in a paleo lifestyle, so help yourself to those and leave the peas on the plate — no matter what your mother used to tell you!

GUT HEALTH

ℓℓℓℓ

You probably don't think about your gut too much, unless you get a tummy bug, but we all know the sense of eating something that 'doesn't agree' with you. Yet gut health is one of the most important aspects of a healthy body, and is coming increasingly into focus in scientific discussion and books about nutrition and health.

The health of your gut determines what nutrients are absorbed and what toxins, allergens and microbes are kept out of your body, and therefore is directly linked to your overall health.

SO, WHAT IS YOUR GUT?

The mouth is the first part of the gut or gastrointestinal tract. When we eat food it passes down the oesophagus and into the stomach, where it gets swished and mulched around a bit with some stomach acid and broken up into the tiniest little pieces. This mush then travels into the small intestine, which is comprised of three sections: the duodenum, jejunum and ileum. The small intestine is where digestion is completed and food is absorbed into the bloodstream.

Following on from the ileum is the first part of the large intestine. The large intestine kind of snakes its way up, across and then down the abdomen, and is where water

THE GUT

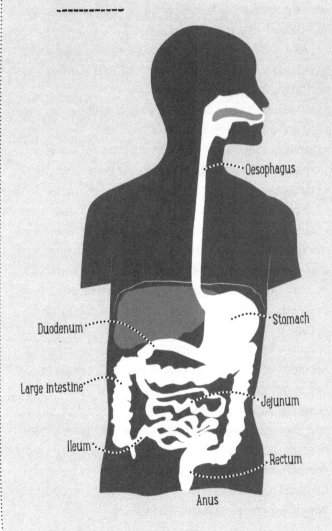

Oesophagus

Duodenum

Stomach

Large intestine

Ileum

Jejunum

Rectum

Anus

is absorbed from the leftover food material. The large intestine carries all of the waste material to the rectum, where it is stored as faeces until it is pushed out through the anus when you go to the toilet.

Your gut is basically the interface between the outside world and your body. It's how food is taken in, absorbed and effectively becomes part of you!

There are two aspects to having a healthy gut: the right mixture of intestinal flora — that is, the micro-organisms that live in your digestive tract — and the barrier between your intestine and your bloodstream and body tissues.

Flora first: your gut contains literally millions of microbes, both good and bad bacteria, which perform a multitude of tasks. The good guys are busy aiding digestion, the absorption of nutrients and your immune system, while the bad guys are just being bad: disrupting processes, causing toxins to build up, and damaging the gut lining.

In an ideal world, your body maintains a natural balance between the good and bad, with the goodies, like in any decent movie, maintaining the upper hand. However, modern lifestyles, including excessive stress and the use of antibiotics, and especially poor-quality modern diets that are high in processed foods, put real pressure on this balance and can let the bad bacteria and funguses like candida (which causes thrush around the body) begin to dominate the scene.

This is where the second aspect comes in to play. If your gut lining is being attacked by bad microbes, it can become inflamed, irritated and even leaky — which is as revolting as it sounds. The gut lining can also be inflamed by eating foods containing gluten and plant foods containing saponins. Once the gut lining is damaged it becomes less efficient as a barrier between your digestive system and the rest of the body. Larger molecules can start to pass through and into your bloodstream, where they are recognised as foreign bodies by the immune system and attacked by your own body. So, basically, there is a little war going on all the time, with your body trying to fight itself.

Another really important aspect of keeping a healthy gut is its effect on your brain. I know they seem a long way apart, but the two areas are intimately connected. We think of the brain as being the home of neurotransmitters like serotonin, which help to control our mood, but in fact our gut is awash with them. More and more scientific studies are showing that the presence or absence of different flora in our gut can alter mood and wellbeing. We talk about having a 'gut feeling' — well, we need to have our gut feeling good!

The good news is that following a paleo lifestyle and avoiding processed foods, sugar and gluten will go a long way towards good gut health. Go easy on your gut — it's the only one you've got, and when it's not working properly you'll know all about it. Be kind to it and it will reward you!

TIP: For the most efficient digestion, make sure you chew your food thoroughly. You have teeth in your mouth, not your stomach. You don't need to chew so much that you get a sore jaw, but ideally chew enough that the food forms a paste-like texture before you swallow.

Chewing your food thoroughly and eating slowly also gives your body's satiety mechanism the chance to kick in — that is, the trigger in your brain that tells you when you've eaten enough food to satisfy your hunger. If you eat too fast then by the time the brain gets this message you've already over-eaten.

ACID VS ALKALINE

Regardless of what a food tastes like, when it is digested and metabolised, it generates either an acid or alkaline effect on the body. Doctors are becoming increasingly aware that this acid-alkaline ratio is vitally important for your health. When this ratio is imbalanced — either too alkaline or too acidic — the body doesn't function very well, and the stage is set for illness and diseases such as arthritis, fibromyalgia, irritable bowel disorders and even cancer to take hold.

Poor dietary habits are the main culprit for causing these imbalances. So knowing and applying this stuff right now may just help to prevent you getting ill — and, at the very least, will help you to feel healthy and full of energy.

In a nutshell, acid-alkaline balance refers to the balance between the amount of acids and non-acids that are found in your body's fluids (blood, saliva and urine) and tissues. This ratio of acids to non-acids is determined by measuring pH levels. pH is measured on a scale of 0 (very acidic) to 14 (very alkaline). A pH of 7 is considered neutral, so a pH level below 7 indicates an acidic condition exists, while a pH level above 7 represents an alkaline condition. The body works at its best when the acid-alkaline balance is slightly alkaline (ideally having a pH of 7.4).

Although this may seem a bit sciency and difficult to apply to your own health, it's actually very simple. All you need to do is be aware of which foods cause an alkaline effect on your body and which cause an acid effect, and try to eat accordingly. There is a more detailed list below, but in general terms foods like cereals and grains, dairy products, meat, eggs, cheese, sugar and salty foods produce an acid load, while fresh fruits and vegetables produce an alkaline load. Don't assume foods will have an acid or alkaline effect based on what they taste like or how much acid they seem to have in them — it's what happens to them when they're digested that matters. For example, lemons, which might seem to be a very acid food, in fact have an alkalising effect once fully metabolised.

Back in the day, our ancestors who followed a paleo lifestyle ate a lot of vegetables and fruits, which would have neutralised the acid load produced by eating meat. They would have been healthier and would have suffered from far fewer illnesses associated with acid–alkaline imbalances. Today, with many people's diets being top-heavy on grains, sugar and dairy, the overall effect on the body is of acid overload — and it's this acid overload that is causing inflammation in the body's tissues and may lead to chronic diseases like cancer. Some people even choose to follow an alkaline-producing foods diet to assist with their cancer treatment.

So it's worth being aware of this stuff if you really want to improve your health. Following are ten easy ways to change your diet slightly to have an alkalising effect on your body.

1. Eat plenty of vegetables, especially leafy green ones.
2. Squeeze some fresh lemon or lime juice into your daily water.
3. Introduce apple cider vinegar to your life — add it to salad dressings or, as I like to do, make a hot water, apple cider vinegar and honey drink first thing in the morning. This will not only have an alkalising effect but will also kick-start your digestive system by boosting stomach acids.
4. Substitute your coffee for green tea once or twice a week.
5. Don't eat too much meat.
6. Reduce your intake of sugary drinks and coffee.
7. Reduce your intake of refined carbohydrates (grains) and sugar.
8. Take a buffered 1000-milligram Vitamin C supplement.
9. Drink lots of water.

10. Combine highly alkaline foods in a meal with foods that are acidic to create better balance and maintain an alkaline pH.

On the following pages you'll find a table that shows you how acid or alkaline many common foods are.

ACID AND ALKALINE FOODS

FOOD CATEGORY	MOST ACID	ACID	LOWEST ACID
SWEETENERS	aspartame	white sugar, brown sugar	processed honey, molasses
FRUIT	blueberries, cranberries, prunes	rhubarb	plums, processed fruit juices
VEGETABLES	—	potatoes (without the skin)	spinach (cooked)
BEANS AND LEGUMES	chocolate, peanuts	pinto beans, lima beans	kidney beans
NUTS AND SEEDS	walnuts	pecans, cashews	pumpkin seeds, sunflower seeds
OILS	—	—	corn oil
GRAINS AND CEREALS	wheat, white flour, pasta	white rice, buckwheat, oats, rye	sprouted wheat bread, spelt, brown rice
MEAT	beef, pork, shellfish	turkey, chicken, lamb	venison, fish
DAIRY	raw milk	eggs, butter, yoghurt, buttermilk, cottage cheese	soy cheese, soy milk, goat's milk, goat's cheese
DRINKS	beer, soft drinks	coffee	tea

| < 5.0 | 5.0 | 5.5 | 6.0 | 6.5 | 7.0 | 7.5 | 8.0 | 8.5 | 9.0 | 9.5+ |

LOWEST ALKALINE	ALKALINE	MOST ALKALINE
raw honey, raw sugar	maple syrup, rice syrup	stevia
oranges, bananas, cherries, pineapple, peaches, avocado	kiwifruit, apples, pears, melons, grapes, dates, figs, raisins	lemons, limes, grapefruit, watermelon, mangoes
carrots, tomatoes, corn (fresh), mushrooms, cabbage, potato skins, olives	beetroot, celery, lettuce, courgettes, kumara	asparagus, spinach (raw), broccoli, parsley, onions, garlic
soybeans, tofu	carob	—
chestnuts	almonds	—
canola oil	flaxseed oil	olive oil
amaranth, millet, wild rice, quinoa	—	—
—	—	—
breast milk	—	—
ginger tea	green tea	herbal teas, lemon water, apple cider vinegar

6. SO WHERE THE HELL DO I BEGIN?

················•

If what you've read so far is making you think, 'Hmmm, maybe it's worth giving this paleo thing a try,' your next thought is probably, 'Where do I start?' For some people it can be a pretty serious revision of the way they eat and their approach to food, but if you have started to take an interest in your health you might find that you are already doing some of these things: staying away from sugar, minimising processed grains, going easy on the beers and so on (see chapter 9 for more on alcohol and other drinks).

There are two ways of getting into the paleo lifestyle: dipping your toe in the water and taking unhealthy foods out of your daily routine one or two at a time, so you don't feel like you are being too deprived; or just going 'cold turkey' and stripping right back to strict paleo basics for a set amount of time — say, a month. That's what I did and, as I have said, once I'd been eating and living this way for a month it was an easy decision to keep on doing it: I felt so good that I had no urge to go back to eating the foods which I had learnt made me feel bad.

There are several advantages to going cold turkey for a month. For a start, that first month acts as a kind of detox: it gives your body a chance to work through what's still in your system and get rid of any lingering toxins. Second, it takes a while for your brain to readjust to what it's not getting (the drug-like effects of sugar consumption, for example). It can take a while for the cravings to wear off, as your brain finally gets used to not getting its regular 'hit'.

Starting off for a fixed amount of time also means you have an end date: on days when you are finding it tough sticking to the lifestyle, you can tell yourself, 'It's only for a month,' or, 'It's only for ten more days,' or whatever, which might help to make your desire to eat that doughnut a little bit easier to bear (and I bet that, at the end of those ten days, you won't even want it any more).

It also gives your taste buds a chance to reset themselves: often they are so swamped with sugars and additives from the processed foods we eat that 'natural' food tastes a bit bland. However, once you have been eating tasty and varied paleo meals for four weeks or so, you'll not only discover how delicious fresh vegetables and fruit, good-quality meat and eggs, fresh nuts and seeds are, but if you do eat something processed it won't taste so good any more.

At the end of the month, you can then loosen up the reins a little bit, if you want. Feel like reintroducing a bit of dairy, perhaps some cheese or a little cream in your coffee? Add it back in. Discovered you can't live without French toast on a Sunday? Let yourself have it. The interesting thing about reintroducing foods is that it's a bit like allergy testing: if you take all the bad things out, then reintroduce them one at a time, you're going to notice pretty quickly which ones make you feel bad. You may not have even realised that these foods made you feel bad; you may have just assumed how you felt was normal.

As I've said, when I started a paleo lifestyle, I did the cold-turkey thing and was really strict for a month. At the end of that time, I decided I wanted to eat some dairy, because I missed cheese and cream in my coffee. That was really all I added back into my diet on a regular basis, and from that time on I have only eaten non-paleo foods very infrequently (probably about 5–10 per cent of the time).

Interestingly, I didn't start on a paleo lifestyle because I thought what I was eating was making me feel bad — I just wanted to try a healthier diet. It wasn't until I stopped eating certain foods that I discovered the effects they had been having on me. I didn't realise that the tiredness I was feeling and the mid-afternoon energy slump were being caused by my diet until I started eating paleo and these symptoms disappeared.

And as time went on I started to notice other things too. I used to get hay fever, at times quite badly, but now I can't even remember the last time I had a runny nose or itchy eyes. I also hardly ever get sick: I think I've had one cold in the last two years — and even that was very mild and lasted only a couple of days.

However, I understand if you don't want to jump straight in with a strict approach from the get-go — that tactic is not for everyone. In that case, maybe work backwards, dropping one bad thing at a time. You might want to start by having a week without breakfast cereal. Then try to go without any bread. After a couple of weeks you might want to cut out sugar or dairy. Keep subtracting until you reach a point you feel comfortable with and you are feeling the benefits of your lifestyle change.

I think the big three to try to cut out first are bread, pasta (if you eat a lot of it) and sugar, plus anything processed that comes in a packet and has ingredients you don't recognise. Look out for numbers or sciency names — chances are these are things you don't want to put in your body.

➤ TIP: I reckon you're doing awesomely well if you are following a paleo lifestyle about 90–95 per cent of the time — that means 18–20 of the 21 meals you eat in a week (breakfast, lunch and dinner each day) should be purely paleo. So that gives you two to four 'opt outs' every week — if you feel like you need to.

Another way to do it is to eat mostly the same foods but *eat less of them*, and more of the good stuff. For example, if you really love potatoes, then go on eating potatoes — just eat fewer, and add a whole lot more leafy green veges to your plate. If you really love sandwiches, maybe try making your sandwiches with just one piece of bread instead of two (like an open sandwich), and then slowly go down to having no bread at all. You don't need to eat less overall, just eat less of the bad stuff.

THREE WAYS OF STARTING PALEO

Here are some examples of charts you could set up for yourself to monitor your progress as you start out on a paleo lifestyle. You could go cold turkey straight away, giving yourself a tick for each day you stick to the paleo template, or a tick for each paleo meal you eat every day. Add it up at the end of the week and see what percentage paleo you have achieved, then test yourself again the next week, for four weeks.

WEEK 1	BREAKFAST	LUNCH	DINNER	SNACKS
MON	✓	✓	✓	X
TUES	✓	✓	X	✓
WED	X	✓	✓	✓
THURS	X	✓	✓	X
FRI	✓	✓	✓	✓

Alternatively, if you want to try to drop foods one or a few at a time, rather than going the whole hog, you might try something like this.

WEEK 1: Cut out all sugar-containing foods.
WEEK 2: Cut out all other processed foods.
WEEK 3: Cut out all grains and high-GI carbohydrates.
WEEK 4: Cut out all dairy.

And if that's too severe, try breaking it into smaller goals.

WEEK 1: Stop eating processed breakfast cereal and have a paleo-friendly breakfast, like poached eggs on spinach, every day.
WEEK 2: Cut down from six coffees a day to two, replacing the others with herbal teas (see chapter 9 for more on coffee and other drinks).
WEEK 3: Reduce the number of days in the week you have sandwiches for lunch from five down to two.

. . . and so on, until you are satisfied that you have eliminated the bad stuff from your diet. (By the way, I reckon that if you start off this way you'll probably gain momentum and want to throw out more and more bad stuff as you go. Try it and see!)

The point is, unless you have a recognised food allergy or intolerance, you can choose which foods you do and don't eat. Paleo is a template: a guideline which I believe, in its strictest form, provides the ideal nutrition for the human body while causing the least amount of inflammation. But you can adapt it however you like. How you approach paleo depends on what your end-goal is: being as healthy as possible, reducing the negative food-related symptoms you are experiencing, losing weight, whatever.

If you're going to live paleo, you need to learn what it means, and the ideas behind it, then try to incorporate that template into your lifestyle without sacrificing too much in the way of your social life and things that you really enjoy. You shouldn't feel constrained by your diet, unable to go out and act normally. That's why paleo is not what you'd traditionally call a 'diet'. Diets generally don't work — or at least aren't sustainable long term — because they are based around an idea of deprivation, and can cause you to feel excluded from regular foods and social activities. A paleo lifestyle enables you to go on doing the things you enjoy without filling your body with unhealthy food.

I think the idea of using paleo as a malleable template works from a psychological point of view — you don't want to feel like you're breaking the rules or doing something wrong when you occasionally eat something that isn't strictly paleo. You've got to enjoy it, and have some flexibility, because that's what makes it sustainable. It's about what you eat *most of the time.*

If I have a not-perfectly-paleo day where I really enjoy eating an almond croissant from a farmer's market and then later go round to my grandparents' for dinner and my grandma has made her incredible gnocchi, I don't beat myself up about it. I think that's OK. If you have a meal out on a Saturday with friends and don't strictly follow paleo rules, but still think about what you're eating and make smart choices, then that's pretty good, especially considering all the great stuff you've eaten throughout the week. You're doing this for you, so give yourself a break. It is also easy to forget how social and emotional eating is, and the impact of this on our mental wellbeing and psychological health.

Unless you have a food allergy or intolerance, or are avoiding a certain food because you know for sure it makes you feel bad (for example, gluten), then paleo is a choice, not an imperative. You choose what you do and don't eat. And sometimes you can choose to eat a food which isn't 'paleo', because it's been made by your grandmother, or you're with friends, or just because *you want to*. It's not a matter of, 'I can't eat X or Y because I have a paleo lifestyle.' It's, 'I choose not to eat this food most of the time, because I want to be as healthy as I can.' Paleo is your choice for health.

You don't want to cut yourself off from other people because of how you eat, nor do you want it to be such a burden that you can't keep it up. You have to make paleo work for you.

Haters gonna hate, and some people are going to give you a hard time about adopting this lifestyle, saying it's a stupid trend or extreme. But who really cares what other people think? This is your body, and you're not

> **➤ TIP**: See page 139 for some good ideas of what's best to eat if you're going out for brunch, lunch or dinner. There are more and more cafés and restaurants around which offer paleo or at the very least gluten-free options, plus you can still enjoy a good steak!

doing this for anyone else — you're doing this because you want to improve your own health. You're the one who feels great and is going to live longer because of it.

Following are some more ways to make your transition to a paleo lifestyle easier and more enjoyable.

GET A SUPPORT TEAM

If you're going to adopt a paleo lifestyle, it helps to have the support of the people around you. It definitely helps if the people you hang out with — be they friends or family — support your decision to eat healthily and look after your body. Keeping control of what you eat is much more difficult when you are around other people — you don't want to look like a weirdo, or make life difficult for your mates by making a fuss about your 'diet' and what you can and can't eat.

It also helps if you have a friend who wants to try the same thing — then you can support each other, go through the experience together and compare notes.

It would have been much harder to try a raw-food diet without the help of my friend Charlotte in Byron Bay, who had been doing it for a while and shared lots of tips and tricks with me. It also made it more enjoyable, spending time with someone who understood and shared my health goals and motivations.

If you want to adopt a paleo lifestyle, it's definitely going to be easier if you are following it with other like-minded people. You might be able to convince your flatmates to give it a try, or some of the people you meet at the gym, or your boyfriend or girlfriend. I'm lucky because most of my friends are health conscious, and at my work, CleanPaleo, most of us follow a paleo lifestyle (though not all of our staff — not yet!), so no one brings in cake for morning tea, and we have a whole warehouse of paleo snacks out the back if we get peckish! We don't have any non-paleo foods in the office, which makes it easier to stay away from temptation during work hours.

CLEAN OUT YOUR PANTRY

And your desk drawer, and your car, and your gym bag, and wherever else you stash food. Self-control is the biggest issue when it comes to eating — and I know this from experience. The best way to avoid 'accidentally' eating non-paleo foods is *to not have them around.* That's right: you can't eat them if you don't have them anywhere near you.

So that means cleaning out your pantry and fridge,

and eliminating any non-paleo-friendly items. Either just chuck them out or cook them all up and invite your friends around for a big 'goodbye to non-paleo' dinner party. Then, so you don't feel deprived, go to the supermarket and stock up on good-quality, natural foods — fresh fruit and veges, eggs, tasty meat, nuts and seeds to snack on.

The other advantage of a pantry overhaul is that it means you'll have all the products on hand to make yourself a variety of yummy paleo meals. Make sure you have plenty of seasonings, herbs, spices and other basics for making delicious sauces and sides. Get some natural, healthy oils to cook with. If it's easy to cook paleo because you have everything you need at hand, you're more likely to stick to it.

Obviously this is more difficult if you live with other people — including your parents — but, if that's the case, make it clear to them what your new lifestyle entails and get them on board to support you. If you can't get them to stop eating sugary snacks, then make sure you're not around when they come out! Go get some exercise or read a book, and know that you are doing your body the bigger favour.

LEAD ME NOT INTO TEMPTATION . . .

You get home from work and there's a big block of chocolate sitting in the fridge that your flatmates have got at the supermarket. It's going to do your head in —

PALEO PANTRY LIST

Here's a list of some basics to have in your pantry and fridge to enable you to whip up tasty paleo meals without having to dash out to the shops every time:

→ Almond/Brazil/cashew or other nut butter
→ Almond flour (for baking)
→ Apple cider vinegar
→ Bacon — free-range and organic if possible
→ Baking soda
→ Balsamic vinegar
→ Cacao powder
→ Canned tomatoes — useful for making sauces
→ Cashews
→ Chicken and vegetable stocks
→ CleanPaleo egg white protein powder
→ Coconut aminos (a soy sauce alternative)
→ Coconut milk or cream
→ Coconut oil
→ Dates
→ Free-range organic eggs
→ Garlic
→ Herbs and spices — get busy with these, to add lots of flavour to your meals
→ Honey
→ Maple syrup
→ Olive oil
→ Onions
→ Salmon (canned or packaged)
→ Sea salt
→ Tuna (canned or packaged)

And of course lots and lots of fresh, seasonal fruit and veges, and good-quality organic meat and poultry.

all you will be able to do is think about it and how you're not supposed to eat it. Would one little nibble really hurt . . . ?

If you find yourself in this situation, and feel your resolve quavering, change the record. Remind yourself why you decided to go down the paleo path, and think about all the good things that have happened to your body and life since you started eating clean. Then get away from the chocolate! Go to the gym, or for a run, hang out with a friend or do something else you enjoy.

FIND SOME NEW FAVOURITE RECIPES

It's harder to stick to a paleo lifestyle if you're always thinking, 'But what am I going to eat now?' Look in this book (see chapter 12), and in other books or online for some great paleo recipes that appeal, and make them part of your repertoire.

Pick a paleo breakfast option that you like. Eggs and fruit are always good, and there are more and more convenient paleo breakfast options on the shelves. (I hear CleanPaleo's range of breakfast blends are pretty damn good . . .) Swot up on some ideas for salads and paleo 'wraps' (using lettuce leaves) for lunches, and find some new favourite dinners.

Some people adopt the philosophy of substituting the foods they can't eat for ones they can, creating paleo versions of meals and foods they used to eat. The classics are pasta, rice and potatoes. The last one is easy — just use kumara instead. And as for pasta and rice, I honestly don't really miss them. I don't tend to make meals in which those components appear to be 'missing'. (I also don't miss them because I don't miss the way they made me feel. Every time I consider eating rice or pasta, I just think about the heavy, slow, tired feeling I am going to get afterwards and, whaddaya know, they don't seem so appetising after that!)

However, if you do feel that you want to replace the texture and practical applications of pasta — soaking up sauce, for example — you can make 'vegetable pasta' from veges like courgettes and carrots (see page 203), or a rice substitute with cauliflower (see page 212). It can be pretty fun experimenting with and making these new dishes. Following are some more suggestions of other simple swap-outs.

BREAD

I find it easier to just not make foods which traditionally require bread, such as sandwiches, but you can either substitute bread or buns for lettuce wraps in lunch options (see page 196), or, if you really feel like bread, try the Paleo Nut and Seed Bread on page 190.

SUGAR

As I've said, artificial sweeteners are no better for you than eating refined sugar. Add sweetness when required with maple syrup (make sure it's the real stuff, not maple-flavoured sugar syrup), dates or honey.

COW'S MILK

If you want a milk alternative on your paleo breakfast blend or for cooking, use a good-quality nut milk, like an almond milk. (By the way, soy milk is out from a paleo point of view, as soybeans are legumes and therefore can cause digestive problems — plus there is also the issue of them containing phytoestrogens, which mimic human hormones and can mix things up a bit in your body.)

VEGETABLE OILS

Swap out canola or other vegetable oils for a good-quality (ideally organic and cold-pressed) coconut oil or olive oil — both are great for cooking and good for you. And, if you don't have an issue with dairy, I recommend cooking with butter for some foods. It just tastes so good, plus it contains little or no lactose.

SOFT DRINKS AND JUICES

Don't go for the diet versions. Just start drinking water. You'll soon get used to the 'taste' — or rather, the lack of it — and start enjoying feeling well hydrated and healthy.

FLOUR

Use a non-grain flour such as tapioca, almond or coconut. Most supermarkets now stock these products in their gluten-free sections.

SOY SAUCE

Try coconut aminos, which is made from fermented coconut sap and salt. It is full of healthy amino acids and doesn't taste coconutty at all, just deliciously savoury.

PEANUT BUTTER

There are other nut butters that are actually made from nuts (not legumes, like peanuts!). Try almond butter (see page 216), Brazil nut butter, cashew butter, or even a combination of all three, called ABC butter.

WILL GOING PALEO MAKE ME LOSE WEIGHT?

This is one of the biggest questions many people have about paleo. For some people it is their main motivation for switching to a paleo lifestyle, whereas others don't want to lose weight and are concerned about the effect it will have.

The short answer is: most probably but not neccesarily. It depends on your body composition when you start and how much you exercise.

For the majority of people, a switch to a paleo lifestyle will result in a loss of body fat. If your reason for adopting a paleo lifestyle is to lose weight, chances are you're eating a lot of processed carbs and sugar and so cutting out that crap and eating real, healthy food will definitely result in weight loss.

However, some people have reservations about starting a paleo lifestyle for fear that they will lose weight and muscle mass, or won't be able to eat sufficient carbs to build muscle. Indeed, I was in this boat before I started. But I soon discovered that wasn't the case at all. I found that I was still able to build muscle, but the most significant thing that happened was that I lost body fat. My overall weight stayed pretty much the same, but my muscle mass increased and my body-fat percentage went down. Muscles love the protein that you get from a paleo diet, and body fat doesn't want to hang around in the absence of starchy carbs and sugar.

The biggest reason your body stores fat is hormonal. By eating paleo and avoiding processed foods containing artificial chemicals, you cut out all those foods which can negatively influence the hormone balance in your body and cause it to store fat, especially in that dangerous area around your waist. (This fat around your waist, the fat that gives people a 'fat gut' look, is called visceral fat. Visceral fat surrounds the vital organs and increases your risk of things like cardiovascular disease, cancers and

Type 2 diabetes.) With paleo, not only are you not eating all that crap in terms of calories, but you are also not giving your body all those toxic substances to deal with.

Most people lose weight initially when they start living paleo, and this is mostly because of a reduction in body fat. Cutting out starchy carbs and processed sugars encourages your body to burn off your fat stores rather than running on carbohydrate. Depending on whether you are currently overweight or at a healthy weight for your height, it might take a while for your body to get used to this new way of eating, but after a while your weight should plateau at a healthy level, and you will find it easy to maintain.

Since I started following a paleo lifestyle, my weight has remained pretty much static. My body-fat percentage has decreased but my body weight seems to have found a set point where it is happy to sit. I believe that everyone's body has a 'set point' where it wants to be — and if you eat what your body was designed to eat, it will naturally revert to this weight and composition. I am able to exercise every day at a high level of intensity, and my body gets all the nutrition it needs to maintain a healthy weight.

Your body's natural set point for weight will vary according to your genetic make-up and there's nothing you can do about that — but give your body the chance to find out what that level is, by eating right and exercising regularly.

A NOTE ON BMI

BMI (body mass index) has been the standard gauge for calculating 'healthy weight' for many years. In fact, the formula (your weight in kilograms divided by the square of your height in metres) was invented by a Belgian doctor in 1832, though our friend Ancel Keys was the one who brought it into wider use (remember him? See page 22). However, BMI is a bit of a blunt instrument.

More recent studies have shown that it's not actually a good gauge of how healthy a person is. For example, you can have a BMI within the 'healthy' range (18.5 to 24.9) but still be carrying an unhealthy amount of visceral fat (remember this is the dangerous fat; see page 124). BMI doesn't provide accurate readings across all ages and ethnicities. And athletes and other fit people who are carrying a significant amount of muscle mass get classified as overweight or even obese. All Blacks captain Richie McCaw, for example, at 1.88 metres tall and around 107 kilograms, is classified as obese. I am 1.89 metres and weigh 93 kilograms, and I am considered overweight using the BMI.

Another rough guide for healthy weight, as indicated by the amount of unhealthy abdominal fat you are carrying, is a waist (circumference) to height ratio. Put simply, the measurement round your waist should be less than half your height, to reduce your risk of obesity-related illness. BMI is an OK way to calculate a rough healthy weight for yourself, but you do need to take other factors into account. If you are serious about getting in the best possible shape, get your body-fat percentage checked at a gym or by your doctor. As a rough guide, a healthy body-fat percentage for men between 20 and 40 years old is between 8 and 19 per cent, with 21–33 per cent considered healthy for women (women have higher body-fat percentages than men because of basic physical differences between the sexes, including hormonal differences).

My body-fat percentage is around 8 per cent, but I don't go around obsessively checking it all the time. If I'm happy with how I look, I'm eating right, I feel good and my clothes fit well, that's good enough for me!

➤ **TIP:** The cells in your body are replaced all the time, and seven years from now every single cell in your body will have been replaced by a completely new one. That means you will have a whole new body — you'll be a whole new person! And what you eat goes into building every one of those millions of cells. You literally are what you eat, because what you put into your body physically creates what you are made of.

Your body wants to make itself the healthiest, strongest body that it can be. It's an unimaginably complex process, but, luckily for you, all you have to do is provide it with the best possible food and your body will do the rest.

7. EATING THE PALEO WAY, DAY TO DAY

·············•

BREAKFAST – THE MOST IMPORTANT MEAL OF THE DAY?

We've all been brought up to believe that you need to have a decent breakfast to set you up for the day. Right from when you're a kid, it's 'Eat your breakfast!' And I used to be just the same: I believed it was the most important meal of the day and ate it religiously every day, without even thinking about whether I was hungry. Until my time in the mining camp, when I started experimenting with different eating regimes and first started fasting (see page 51), I had never challenged the idea of eating breakfast.

Breakfast in Western societies is usually carb-heavy. (Some European cultures, like the Germans, have sausages and other deli meats with breakfast, but there's still too many starchy carbs.) Unless you are a farmer or manual worker and having a cooked breakfast every morning — like shearers who would have mutton chops for breakfast — then you are probably used to having some sort of grain for breakfast, usually cereal and/or toast.

Most manufactured cereals are heavy in carbs, full of sugar and often have little nutritional value. Nutri-Grain, which is promoted as being the breakfast cereal for athletes, is 32 per cent sugar — that's about 8 teaspoons in a 100-gram serving! Weet-Bix are only 2.8 per cent sugar (less than a teaspoon in 100 grams), but that's before you put the sugar on them . . . Plus you usually have your cereal with lactose-rich dairy products, like milk or yoghurt. Then the toast: high-GI bread, usually spread with something sugary like honey, jam, marmalade or Nutella. By starting the day with high-GI carbohydrates, you are setting yourself up for swinging blood sugar levels and fluctuating energy throughout the day.

It's unlikely that our ancestors ate anything for breakfast — generally they ate when they had food, and they certainly weren't sitting around the fire sucking up porridge. Hell, even the Romans didn't eat breakfast. It wasn't until around the 1700s that the wealthy started having a special morning meal, and not until the Industrial Revolution that most people ate something before heading off to the factory for the day. Eating pre-prepared cereal for breakfast only became a thing after the Kellogg brothers accidentally invented the cornflake in 1898 — then proceeded to sell it to us like we'd been missing it throughout the course of human evolution!

Breakfast has been made into what it is by marketing: big companies telling you how to start the day 'right' by consuming their products. It has been turned into a supermarket category, and there is often a whole aisle dedicated to the stuff. What we know as 'breakfast' has been created by big companies in order to sell boxes of cheap-to-produce grains and sugar — marketed in a way that makes people believe they are making a 'healthy' choice.

I personally don't eat breakfast, unless I am exercising first thing in the morning (and, even then, I don't usually eat until afterwards). At first I thought I missed it, but once I started listening to my body and eating paleo I found that I wasn't waking up feeling hungry, and was happy to go through till lunchtime without eating most days.

I think that, for most people, breakfast is something you only need to eat if you're actually hungry (like all meals). Don't assume that just because you've woken up and it's the morning you need to eat something. Think about what your body is telling you. Are you actually gagging for something to eat, or just fulfilling a habit, which involves necking an instant coffee and a bowl of cereal before running out the door to work?

(It's important to note, though, that just because you don't have breakfast doesn't mean you should snack all day until it's time to have a 'decent' meal at lunchtime.

If you're hungry in the mornings, eat a healthy, paleo breakfast. If you're not, wait until your body is sending you hunger signals; by all means have a sensible snack, then eat a well-balanced, nutritious lunch. You might be surprised at how you can retrain yourself to not eat automatically as soon as you get up in the morning.)

BUT WHAT IF I DO WANT BREAKFAST?

Having said all that, I understand that some people do still want or feel that they need breakfast. So what can you eat in the mornings if you are living a paleo lifestyle?

The most simple option is, of course, fruit. As discussed above, most manufactured breakfast cereals are not paleo, so they're out (see the box on page 133 about paleo 'breakfast blends'). If you do find that you genuinely are really hungry in the morning or feel that you require a large breakfast to keep you going with physical work on which you will be expending a lot of energy, then a cooked breakfast is a good way to go. Eggs, bacon and avocado is a good option. Or make yourself an omelette with veges in it. (See why I love eggs? They really do come in handy.)

At weekends I sometimes make paleo pancakes out of bananas and eggs (see page 189), and serve them with maple syrup. The first time I experimented with them I thought they would be terrible because the combination sounded a bit odd, but they're actually better than normal pancakes (and a million times healthier).

WHAT IF I'M OUT FOR BRUNCH?

Going out for brunch is one of life's pleasures, and is often more about the social side of catching up with friends and family than the actual food. But every time I go out to a café I notice that the first three things on the menu are usually a cereal (often a muesli or granola), something to do with toast or bagels, and pancakes — i.e. nothing paleo! Down the list you'll get into the eggs-and-bacon department, and there are usually a few more compatible options, but often it takes some tweaking to get it right — especially weeding out the toast toast toast that seems to come with everything!

I'll often order the bacon and eggs or the cooked breakfast, or even the eggs Benedict and just make sure I ask for them without any non-paleo foods, like toast, bagels or hash browns. A lot of cafés offer great omelettes, which get the tick as well.

More and more cafés are offering paleo options, and in the bigger cities there are places opening up where the whole menu is paleo. (Google 'paleo cafés' in your area to find out who's offering the good stuff.) Suggest to your friends that you meet up at one of these and *bam!* You don't have to struggle with the menu at all. You might even convert a few of your friends along the way!

And, remember also — following a paleo lifestyle doesn't necessarily mean eating clean every second of every day. If you go out for brunch every so often and end up eating something you wouldn't normally, it's not the end of the world. As long as you are trying to eat healthily most of the time, your body will thank you for it.

If you're out and about, or having lunch with colleagues or as a business meeting, many cafés now offer a paleo option — or, at least, a gluten-free option which might also be close to paleo. Order a salad or vege dish, or order a steak sandwich or burger and ask them to hold the bread. Also ask for no sauce, or have it on the side so you can just have a little if it's super tasty. (Barbecue sauce in particular is often full of sugar. We're talking more than three times as much sugar as Coke!)

Sushi, which is a popular and easy lunch choice for many people, is an interesting one. Strictly speaking, sushi is not paleo — as well as the rice itself, it usually has sugar added as flavouring. However, the amount of rice in each slice of sushi is quite low, especially if there is lots of tasty protein and vegetable filling. So make your own choice. Sashimi — slices of raw fish — is a safe paleo choice, as are some other items on the Japanese menu (see page 142) but watch out for the soy sauce.

DINNER TIME!

You've finished a hard day's work, headed to the gym or for a run, and now you're hanging out for dinner. So what's on the paleo menu?

If you were brought up in the average Kiwi household, most of your dinners growing up probably involved meat paired with either potatoes, rice, noodles or pasta and with a small portion of some sort of vegetables on the side. We're a nation of meat eaters — we eat three times the world average amount of meat per head each year — which is great from a paleo point of view, as long as that meat is fresh, grass-fed and organic if possible. But it's the question of what goes with that meat that can be a bit confounding if you're living a paleo lifestyle. We are so used to the easy, quick carbohydrate items, and to eating ethnic foods which are often also based around starchy carbs like rice or noodles, that it can require a bit of a mindset change to rejig our dinner menu.

The great news is you won't be going without. The abundance of fresh, healthy, seasonal vegetables in New Zealand means you will always have plenty on your plate, without having to 'make up for' the missing starchy carbs. Not eating potatoes, rice, pasta or noodles doesn't mean you have to eat more meat. If you include plenty of different veges in your meals you will feel full and satisfied — and full of energy.

I personally find dinner an easy paleo meal — a lot of what you probably eat already fits into a paleo lifestyle, with a few tweaks. Just think 'meat and three vege'. Back in the old days, one of those veges would probably have been potatoes, but swap those out for kumara, and add a tasty salad or some carrots and broccoli (or whatever your favourite veges are) to your meat or fish selection and you're done.

Your protein options are pretty broad: grass-fed beef and lamb and free-range pork if you're into red meat; free-range, organic chicken, duck or turkey, and fresh-caught white fish or salmon. If you can get good-quality sausages made by your local butcher that contain mostly or only meat (you can get some great gluten-free ones), then go for it! I love saussies and think they are so underrated. If you're choosing bacon, make sure it's cruelty-free and free-range too. Check to see if your butcher makes their own bacon — a lot of what you buy in the supermarket has sugar and nitrates (preservatives) added to it, not to mention quite a lot of water.

As I've already said, I usually shop every day or two to make sure everything is fresh, choosing whatever meat looks good or is on special then basing my evening meal around that. I usually pick at least three different veges — again, choosing what's in season, on special or will go well with the dish — or I make a big salad, with as many different leaves and veges in it as possible, and throw in some chopped nuts or hard-boiled egg to keep it exciting. Sometimes I make a simple sauce, but mostly I eat my meat pretty plain — good-quality meat is so tasty on its own, it doesn't need disguising! I also try to keep my cooking pretty simple, as I don't have much time at the end of the day to spend hours in the kitchen, but if that's your thing you can be a lot more creative and have a lot of fun.

I have a few favourite go-to recipes: Paleo Burgers (see page 199) and courgette 'pasta' (see page 203) especially, and I love making myself a big salad and adding some chicken or beef strips to make it really hearty. I usually have fish once or twice a week — either salmon or paleo fish and chips (see page 207) — and once a week I might have a meat-free meal — something like a veges-only stir-fry, or something made from eggs. Soups are also good, especially in winter, and you can make a big batch and freeze portions to eat later (see pages 197–198).

If you really miss the texture and practicality of pasta (let's be honest, it doesn't have much taste, so it's the pasta-eating experience you're missing) you can make courgette spaghetti (or 'courgetti', if you will) by cutting long strips of 'pasta' from the outside of a courgette (see page 203 for more on this). Carrots and parsnips can be prepared this way too.

I have included some of my favourite recipes in chapter 12. Go online for heaps more inspiration — google 'paleo recipes' and you will be spoilt for choice.

ANYONE FOR DESSERT?

I love dessert. I especially love chocolate. There are some great low-sugar, high-cocoa-solids chocolates available (I'm talking about the dark chocolates that say 70–80 per cent on them), so every now and then I will treat myself to a few squares after dinner.

If I'm eating out, I will have dessert sometimes, as part of my 5–10 per cent of meals that aren't paleo. You'd be hard pressed to find a paleo dessert on a restaurant menu, so I just pick something that sounds really, really nice and eat it without feeling guilty. So there!

There are also a lot of interesting and delicious paleo desserts that you can make at home, usually using dates, honey, maple syrup or fruit as a sweetener. Just jump online and have a look at all of the ideas and recipes for things like paleo cookies, brownies, fruit treats and puddings.

WHAT IF I'M GOING OUT?

Maintaining a paleo lifestyle is much easier if you are preparing and cooking all your own food. Then you know where it's come from, and what's gone into it. However, you can't live like a hermit! If you're going to be eating out at a non-paleo eatery, you really have only one option: make it one of your non-paleo meals for the week, but still make smart choices. Remember, eating should be a pleasurable experience, not a minefield.

Here are some tips to make it easier.

→ Try to choose foods which are at least close to your usual paleo diet — meat and plenty of vegetables.

→ Don't go crazy on the carbs. If you're having Indian, Thai or Chinese, have some rice — but not heaps. Don't be tempted by the bread basket.

→ Don't overeat — we all tend to eat more with other people, but it's no excuse to totally pig out. If you are getting full but still have food on your plate, just leave it. The fact that you have paid for it doesn't mean you have to finish it — you'll pay the same amount regardless of whether you stuff yourself and feel sick or eat only as much as you need to and leave feeling perfectly full and comfortable.

→ Ask for sauces on the side.

→ Don't be afraid to ask for tweaks to the menu —
  if you want to remove or swap out one or two
  ingredients (like replacing potatoes with kumara
  or more of another vegetable, or switching fries for
  vegetables, or holding a sauce or cheesy topping),
  just ask. The worst thing a waiter can say is no
  (and, remember, at any place with decent service,
  the customer is always right!).
→ Look for the gluten-free options on the menu. Often
  they won't be strictly paleo, but they will obviously
  be gluten free and hopefully a healthier choice.
  (By the way, I reckon that in five or ten years it'll
  be common to see a little symbol showing which
  dishes on a menu are paleo, just like we see with
  'vegetarian' and 'gluten-free' symbols now. Then
  things will be a bit easier!)
→ Don't get stressed about what you're eating and
  what might be in it. Chances are, anything that's
  been prepared in a restaurant is going to have
  something non-paleo in it, even if it's just the
  canola oil the food's been cooked in. Sitting there
  with your friends and saying you can't eat anything
  is just going to make you look and feel like a chump.
  Be mindful of what you order, but not obsessive,
  and stick to your usual healthy routine the rest of
  the time.

ETHNIC RESTAURANTS

In New Zealand, we are lucky to have such a huge range of different cuisines on offer. It can be a bit difficult to work out what the best paleo choices are when eating out in an ethnic restaurant, though, so here are some tips.

➳ THAI, VIETNAMESE AND SIMILAR ➳

As long as you don't overdo it on the rice, Thai and Vietnamese restaurants can offer some decent paleo choices.

Avoid: dishes with rice or noodles, soy sauce, sweet chilli sauce.

Best options: whole baked or poached fish, papaya salad, hotpot (where you simmer meat and veges in a broth), stir-fried veges, larb, beef salad, seafood salad, tom yum soup, meat and vegetable curries.

➳ CHINESE ➳

Ordering Chinese food when out can be really difficult, as there are so many sauces, flavourings and additives. Try to keep it simple.

Avoid: dishes with rice or noodles, MSG, soy sauce, sweet-and-sour sauce, oyster sauce, anything deep fried.

Best options: meat and vege stir-fries, steamed veges.

JAPANESE

My favourite ethnic food. Again, go easy on the rice and enjoy the lovely fresh flavours.

Avoid: rice or noodles (although buckwheat and soba noodles are at least gluten free), tempura and other deep-fried dishes, tofu (which is made from soybeans).

Best options: sashimi, seaweed salad, steamed vegetables (they do great things with broccoli!), beef tataki, grilled chicken or salmon, yakitori, shabu-shabu (meat and veges you cook in broth), omelettes.

ITALIAN

Just because you're eating at an Italian restaurant doesn't mean you have to go mad on the pasta and pizza. Italians, in fact, eat only small amounts of it, as a precursor to their main dish, which is usually — wait for it — meat and vegetables or salad. And Italians wouldn't dream of eating what passes for pizza outside Italy!

Avoid: pasta, pizza, bread.

Best options: antipasti, grilled meat or fish with vegetables.

MEXICAN

Another difficult one, as much Mexican food comes wrapped in a flour- or corn-based shell, and is often served with rice or refried beans. However, the Mexicali Fresh chain has a paleo salad option which is worth checking out, and you can still find good tasty options.

Avoid: tortillas, corn chips, burritos, taco shells, cheesiness.

Best options: meat, salad, salsa, guacamole, ceviche, plus fajitas are a good option if you leave out the tortilla wraps.

‑◦ INDIAN ◦‑

Very difficult. Basically, very little Indian food is paleo. My recommendation is, if you feel like having a curry, have a curry. Enjoy it. But don't kid yourself. Get back on the paleo wagon the next day.

‑◦ MIDDLE EASTERN ◦‑

There can be some really good, tasty paleo options at a Turkish or Middle Eastern restaurant.

Avoid: hummus (which is made from chickpeas), pita bread, yoghurt sauces, rice.

Best options: grilled and roasted meats, shish kebabs, grilled veges, salads.

‑◦ SPANISH/TAPAS ◦‑

Small plates with intense flavour and usually cooked with healthy olive oil, tapas can be a good choice.

Avoid: breads, potato dishes, paella, churros.

Best options: calamari, meat skewers, meatballs, prawns and squid, cured meats, vege dishes.

8. PALEO ON THE GO
WHAT'S OK TO SNACK ON

...............•

I personally get by on three, often two, meals a day, if I am intermittently fasting — and that's it. That might seem like not very much food if you are used to the 'little and often' eating pattern, or if you are in the habit of enjoying morning and afternoon tea, and sometimes supper, which brings you up to six meals a day. But I have found that my body has got used to this level and pattern of nutrition. Because my blood sugars are stable due to the foods I eat (and because they are no longer being affected by the high-GI foods I have cut out of my diet), I no longer get energy and concentration slumps or feel the urge to have a wee snack to get me going again.

However, while I don't get sugar cravings, there are certainly times when I need to eat a little something to keep me going until my next major meal; and I do like to eat after a workout.

Basically, there are very few packaged snacks which tick the paleo box. Most muesli or snack-type bars are obviously not going to fit the lifestyle, and even things like 'healthy' nut bars are usually packed with sugar. It's actually quite worrying that these sugary muesli bars are so heavily marketed as healthy snacks for kids.

Here are some healthy paleo snack ideas.

→ **Fresh fruit.** Sweet, tasty, satisfying and totally paleo. Just don't go overboard — it still contains sugar, even if it is natural, so don't eat too much. My personal favourite is bananas — a really great low-GI snack, they are also a great source of potassium, vitamin B6, sterols (a healthy fat) and dietary fibre. Watch out for dried fruit — you wouldn't eat five apricots at once, so don't eat five dried ones. I personally try to have only two pieces of fruit a day.

→ **Dates.** If you're looking for a sweet hit that's totally natural and delicious, you can't go past fresh dates. Again, just have one or two — they are super sweet and I'll bet you won't be able to eat more than two at a time anyway!

→ **Vegetable crudités (or sticks).** Carrots, celery, broccoli, cauliflower, capsicum, mushrooms — whatever tickles your fancy, cut it into small chunks and keep it handy in the fridge for quick snacks. If you want to jazz them up, dip them in some guacamole or home-made salsa.

→ **Nuts.** A small handful of nuts will give you a burst of sustained energy, help to sharpen your mind and provide nutrients such as calcium, iron, magnesium and selenium.

→ **Biltong.** You might not have tried this before, but dried meat is a great paleo snack. CleanPaleo produces a grass-fed, air-dried beef biltong snack, seasoned with a little salt, pepper and coriander, which is totally delicious. You can also just snack on regular cold meat, if you have some roast left over.

→ **Hard-boiled eggs.** Boil up a few at a time and keep them in the fridge for a quick protein snack. So handy.

→ **Tinned fish.** Those little cans or sachets of tuna or salmon aren't just for feeding the cat — they make a great snack. The flavoured ones contain a few additives and sugar, so stick to fish packed in spring water or olive oil.

→ **Herbal teas.** Sometimes a refreshing cup of peppermint or other herbal tea is enough of a boost without eating as well.

→ Another snack that CleanPaleo makes are **CoGo Bites**, which are little bursts of flavour! They are made from natural fruit juices and purées combined with organic coconut milk and freeze-dried. They're just the right combination of crunchy and melt-in-your-mouth. Mmmm . . .

Keep a few of these options handy and you'll never be tempted by a quick fix from the gas station or dairy.

WHY DO WE SNACK?

The reasons we snack aren't as straightforward as just fulfilling a biological need for energy between larger meals. Often, we reach for food for psychological reasons: we're bored; we need something to do with our hands; we're feeling sad or tired; other people are eating around us or have offered us something; or it's staring at us from the fridge and we can't think of a good enough excuse not to eat it! Like eating breakfast, or having certain foods at set mealtimes, sometimes we eat just because we think we are hungry, or because it's 'time' for food. So, if you've got a bit of a snack habit, the first thing you need to do is think about why you snack.

If you take a look at it — maybe jot down what you're eating over the course of a few days, and when — you might see some patterns emerging. Do you always eat morning tea, because that's when everyone in your work team stops and has a cup of tea? Do you find yourself reaching for chocolate at around 3pm, after the effects of your carbohydrate-laden lunch are making themselves felt? Do you grab something at the gas station when filling up the car, because there's usually a good special on?

If you stop to consider whether you are actually hungry and need food at these times, you might find that you can knock your snacking on the head. Also, once you have adopted a paleo lifestyle you will probably find that eating three quality meals a day made from natural, wholefood ingredients, without any of the bad stuff, fills you up and gives you plenty of energy without having to 'top up' in between.

FOOD AS A REWARD

Another mental hurdle I think we need to get over is the idea of food being a 'reward' (or, in some cases, having something to eat to make up for something bad happening, like a tough meeting or an argument with a friend). I think this starts in childhood, when we are given 'treats' for behaving ourselves, like ice cream or lollies. If we are brave and don't cry when we have an injection at the doctor, we get given food. If we eat all our dinner, we get dessert. If we don't hit our sister in the back of the car, we stop for an ice cream.

I'm not saying you shouldn't do this (although if you're a parent it's worth thinking about the long-term implications), but it's something that we need to get over as adults. Now we are in control of the food supply, we can choose what we eat, and for what reasons. And we can choose how we reward ourselves — or cheer ourselves up — with things other than food.

My favourite pick-me-up is exercise. If I've had a bad

day at work, or I'm feeling stressed out for personal reasons, I hit the gym or go for a run. Getting the blood and the endorphins flowing, thinking about my workout rather than my problems, and getting the satisfaction of meeting a challenge all get my head back in the right space. Likewise, because I enjoy the buzz I get from exercise, I see that as a reward too.

For you, it might be a yoga class, some time reading a book or magazine, meeting up with friends, a walk on the beach or watching a favourite movie or TV programme. Whatever makes you feel good!

9. DRINKS

COFFEE — THE GOOD AND THE BAD

Google 'is coffee paleo?' and you come up with a range of answers. Obviously the espressos we drink now are not something our ancestors were drinking, but on the face of it coffee doesn't go against the paleo template: it isn't sugary or highly processed, it's not a starchy carbohydrate and it doesn't contain gluten. And, of course, most of us are, if not addicted to it, at least very strongly attached — myself included. Of course, I'm talking real coffee here: none of this sugary coffee-flavoured milk crap.

I'm not going to tell you how to drink your coffee, but if you want to be as paleo as possible then you should be taking it black. If you really don't like it black, or like a change every now and then like me, try adding a splash of runny cream. (Cream is less processed than milk and doesn't contain as much lactose — remember, lactose is a sugar and the thing that upsets some people's tummies. In my opinion, cream is more delicious too.)

Paleo guru Dr Loren Cordain says if you're going to be strictly paleo you need to lay off the brown stuff, while more moderate thinkers say it's OK in small quantities. It's the caffeine that's the issue: sure, it wakes us up and makes us feel more alert, energetic and happy, but it can also have negative effects on the body, which I'll outline below. Personally, I only drink a maximum of two coffees a day, usually black, but sometimes with a little bit of cream. I also try to use the best-quality organic coffee I can. Luckily there are lots of great local roasters producing very high-quality organic coffees in New Zealand.

Another option I have tried is Bulletproof Coffee — the original recipe is actually a registered trademark but the basic combination is a long black (a double shot of coffee) with a teaspoon of unsalted butter (you must use unsalted as salted makes it taste pretty shit — trust me) and a teaspoon of coconut oil or MCT (medium-chain triglyceride) oil added. (MCTs are a special kind of fat processed from coconut oil which are digested more easily then regular long-chain triglyceride fats.) I know, it sounds disgusting, but just try it and you'll be amazed. It took me two or three to get used to the taste but now I love it — a bit like when you first start drinking your coffee black. The effect of the oils and fats acting on your body and brain along with the caffeine wakes you up heaps more than a 'straight' coffee does.

Coffee can also be useful as a performance-enhancing substance before a gym workout or other physical activity. You might not get any actual additional energy from it from a nutritional point of view, but the way it acts on the brain means you have a sense of having more energy and feel more alert and focused on your workout. It can make you feel more positive.

Coffee works on the brain by stimulating the release of the neurotransmitter dopamine — in the same way that drugs like cocaine and ecstasy do, just in a socially acceptable, legally available way! Unfortunately, the more coffee we drink the better our liver gets at detoxifying it, and we end up needing more and more to get the same high.

And that brings me to the negative effects. Consuming caffeine leads to an elevation in stress hormones, which can cause a bit of havoc in your body and mess with your metabolism — especially if you are drinking a lot of it (more than four cups a day). These stress hormones, including cortisol, make it more difficult for you to lose weight — when we are stressed our body goes into survival mode and stops burning fat.

Coffee also has an acid effect on your body (refer back to page 102 for more info on this), and can cause inflammation to your body tissue.

Because of its lovely psychoactive properties, caffeine is also addictive. After the nice high, you can find yourself having coffee 'lows', and the only way to fix them is to drink more coffee — similar to blood-sugar spikes and dips.

And, of course, if you drink it too late in the day

those wide-awake qualities you enjoy first thing in the morning won't be so attractive when you are trying to get to sleep at 11pm. I personally never drink coffee after 3pm. Caffeine has a half-life of nearly six hours, meaning it takes your body that amount of time to break down half the amount of caffeine you have consumed. And not everyone's body is the same: some people are more sensitive to caffeine than others, and their livers take longer to process it. You probably know your own level of what is just right and what is too much (even if you don't want to admit it to yourself!).

If you feel like your coffee consumption is getting out of hand, or has become a serious crutch to get you out of bed and keep you going throughout the day, try going on a caffeine detox. Go cold turkey for a few days, a week or longer even, and see how you feel. If you then want to go back to drinking it, go ahead — your liver has probably appreciated the break. If you find you're not missing it or that herbal tea is a good substitute, then great. (Just remember, if you have swapped it for green tea, that still contains caffeine. And if you've simply switched to drinking decaf, why bother drinking coffee at all? They usually make decaf by rinsing the coffee beans in a solvent. Still want to drink it?)

I recently gave up coffee for Dry July (a fundraiser where people usually give up alcohol for the month in support of adults living with cancer) — not because I think it is bad for me, but because I wanted to prove it didn't have such a grip on me that I couldn't stop drinking it if I wanted to. I wanted to free myself from

its dark brown tentacles wrapped round my neck . . .
anyway, it was a long month, and I think I missed the
social aspect of having a coffee more than the drug
itself, but I made it. I'd like to cut down to one cup a day
too, but let's not rush into things . . .

TEAS

I'm a great fan of a decent cup of tea. Black tea contains
antioxidants, and green tea is even better for you —
because it is less processed, it contains even more
good stuff, and has been shown to have health benefits
ranging from lowering cholesterol and blood pressure
to reducing the incidence of Alzheimer's disease and
improving your memory. Teas are also fantastic for
your digestive system.

Green tea does contain caffeine, but less than black
tea does and certainly less than coffee. So it provides
a mild pick-me-up effect without being as addictive or
giving you the shakes if you have too much of it!

My other favourites are:
→ peppermint tea — cleansing and good for digestion
→ chamomile — calms and relaxes you
→ liquorice — relaxing and anti-inflammatory.

ALCOHOL

The big question. In short: no, alcohol is not compatible with a paleo lifestyle. There, have you heard enough?

However . . . while drinking alcohol doesn't fit in with a strict paleo diet — it's both a processed food and a toxin, and our ancestors certainly weren't drinking it — it is, for better or worse, a major part of our culture. And I'm not just talking about the Kiwi binge-drinking culture — I mean our social lives, our gatherings, our ways to relax and spend time with friends. Giving up drinking entirely is a personal decision and a pretty big call — although, if you want to do that, I admire that decision. You will almost certainly be better off because of it.

But, if going completely dry doesn't appeal, what are the best options if you're trying to live a paleo lifestyle?

Interestingly, besides the macronutrients protein, fat and carbohydrate, alcohol is the only other substance that can provide calories (energy) to the body — it is not classified as a macronutrient, however, because it is not essential for survival and doesn't contain any valuable micronutrients. But, gram for gram, alcohol provides nearly twice as much energy as protein or carbohydrate. This means that when you are enjoying an alcoholic beverage you are not only consuming the carbohydrates and sugars it contains, but also the energy provided directly by the alcohol. And, unless you're cutting some mad shapes on the dance floor, chances are you're not expending that extra energy.

Another side effect is that, because alcohol is

effectively a toxin, your liver views breaking it down and getting rid of it as a number-one priority — so it stops doing all the other things it needs to do while it works on that project. That means the digestion and metabolism of any food (especially fat) you have eaten is going to be sidelined while your liver is otherwise engaged. That basically means that, while your body is metabolising the alcohol, you will be storing fat instead of burning it.

Personally, I do drink some alcohol, but not that often. When I do, I usually go for a red wine or a white spirit — vodka or gin — with soda water, a squeeze of lemon and some cucumber. Other mixers are out; even tonic water has sugar in it (around 9 grams per 100 millilitres!). Every now and then, if I'm having a special night out, I am rather partial to espresso martinis (vodka, coffee liqueur and a shot of espresso).

My other option is red wine. Some studies suggest the antioxidants and a substance called resveratrol which it contains have health benefits when consumed in moderation. Also, I like red wine because it is the closest thing to a 'natural' or traditional form of alcohol which has been enjoyed for thousands of years.

And of course there's beer. So refreshing after a long day's work. The problem is it's anything but refreshing for your body, with its poisonous trifecta of alcohol, sugar and gluten. One every now and then is OK, but drinking it every day will do seriously bad things to your health. Don't shoot the messenger — I'm just giving it to you straight.

My personal preference is to have two or three drinks

on that one night a week when I drink, rather than drinking alcohol every day. That gives my liver plenty of time to completely detox between 'doses'.

HOW CAN I STAY HYDRATED?

The most important issue when talking about what to drink is staying hydrated. And, of course, the simplest way to achieve this is by drinking plenty of water. Nothing fancy, no additives: just plain old tap water.

A lot of everyday ailments that people experience — like headaches, energy dips and tiredness — are caused by dehydration, and can be avoided by drinking enough water.

I try to drink about 3 litres of water a day, which sounds like a lot, but if you drink little swigs often you can easily get through it. Carry a drink bottle with you and sip on it regularly. I'm aware of all of the negatives associated with plastic bottles so I like to drink out of glass bottles and refill them. I also think water just tastes better out of glass.

The only times I don't drink water are 30 minutes before and 30 minutes after eating, as water dilutes the acid in your stomach and makes digestion less efficient.

And even if you're training — unless you're in the All Blacks or a pretty serious athlete or runner — you don't need sports drinks. Many of them contain sugar (often by another name) and are little better than soft drinks. Stick with healthy water.

ELECTROLYTES

You might have seen the term 'electrolytes' thrown around when it comes to sports drinks. Electrolytes are minerals carried in your blood and other bodily fluids which help to regulate bodily processes such as the acidity of your blood, your hydration level and muscle function. They include potassium, sodium, magnesium and phosphorus. If you work out hard and sweat a lot but don't replace these minerals you might find your muscles starting to cramp up — that's a sign your electrolyte level has been depleted.

If you are sweating a lot, drinking water alone will not replenish these minerals. But that doesn't mean you have to pay $4.50 for a bottle of coloured water with sugar in it!

If I am exercising a lot and know I am going to be sweating — and therefore excreting minerals and salts through my skin — I will eat a banana. They are high in available energy, high in good carbohydrates and contain minerals such as magnesium and potassium. Eating a banana is just as efficient as and much more economical than having a sports drink or carb shot. I work out at a very high intensity and sweat a lot, but I never get cramps, so that tells me my electrolyte levels are fine.

Unless you are an elite athlete training at a very high level, you don't need sports drinks. For many people they are just an excuse to get a sugary hit. End of story.

➤ TIP: A lot of the 'exercise food' industry — protein powders, sports drinks, nutrition bars and so on — is just marketing. If you're a normal person trying to be as healthy as you can and doing a moderate amount of regular exercise, you don't really need anything extra in your diet other than what we've been talking about: lean meat, lots of vegetables and fruit, healthy fats, nuts, seeds and lots of water.

10. NUTRITION AND EXERCISE
WHAT DO I NEED TO EAT?

· · · · · · · · · · · · · · ●

While healthy eating is a huge part of the paleo lifestyle, getting plenty of exercise is a really important component too, as we'll look at in the second section of this book. Exercise and nutrition are linked: there's no point in doing heaps of exercise but still eating badly, or eating really well but not giving your body the exercise it needs to function at its best. But the big mistake that many people make is thinking that because they are exercising they automatically need to eat more or eat differently. Wrong! As we will discuss in the next section, the human body is designed to move and be used for physical exercise, and it doesn't necessarily need to be fed anything fancier than a clean, nutritious

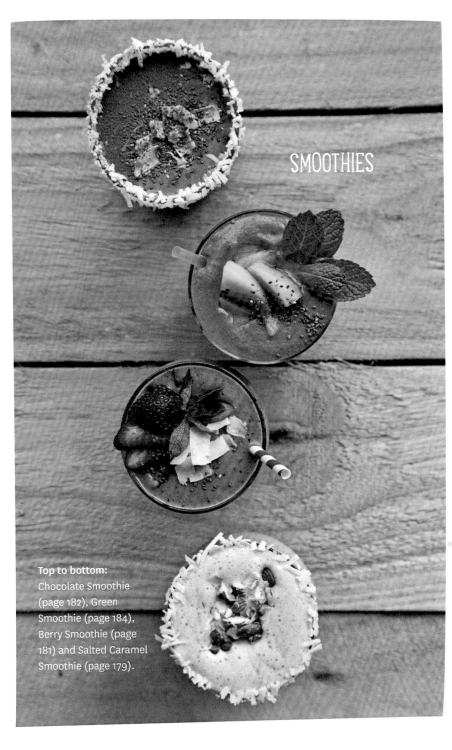

SMOOTHIES

Top to bottom:
Chocolate Smoothie
(page 182), Green
Smoothie (page 184),
Berry Smoothie (page
181) and Salted Caramel
Smoothie (page 179).

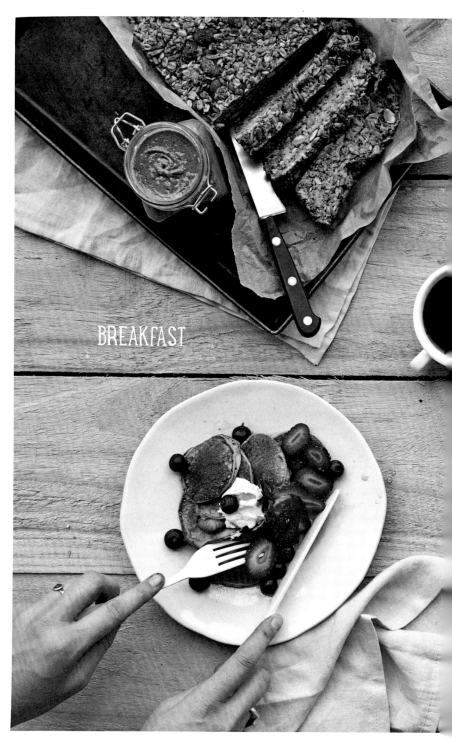

BREAKFAST

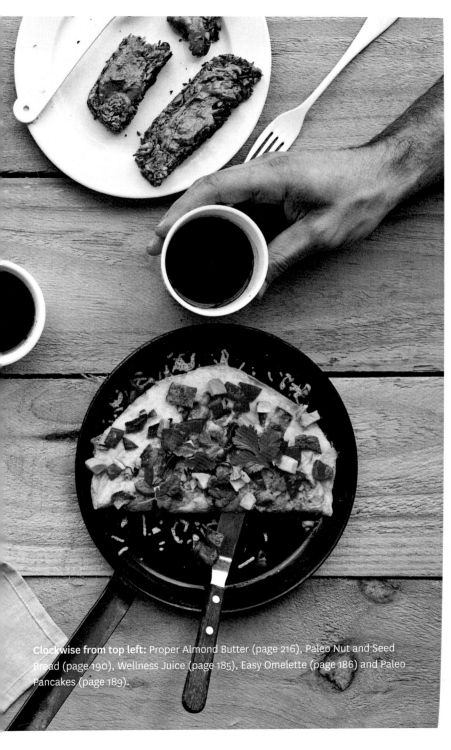

Clockwise from top left: Proper Almond Butter (page 216), Paleo Nut and Seed Bread (page 190), Wellness Juice (page 185), Easy Omelette (page 186) and Paleo Pancakes (page 189).

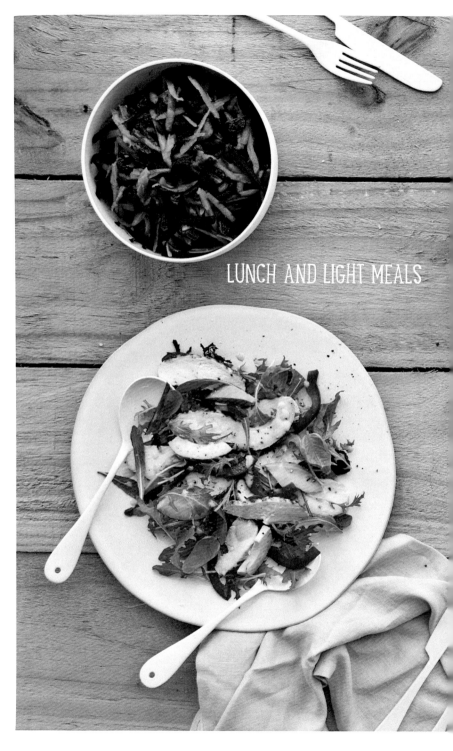

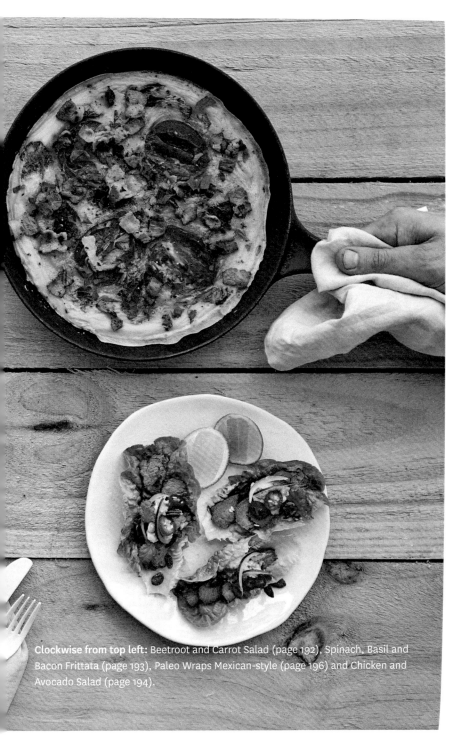

Clockwise from top left: Beetroot and Carrot Salad (page 192), Spinach, Basil and Bacon Frittata (page 193), Paleo Wraps Mexican-style (page 196) and Chicken and Avocado Salad (page 194).

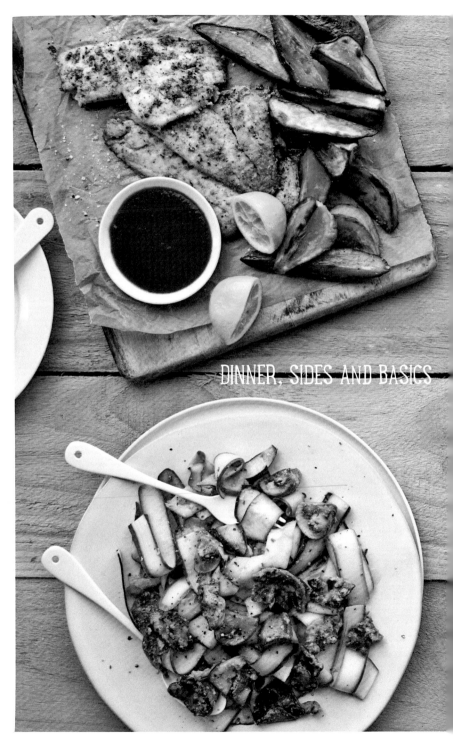

DINNER, SIDES AND BASICS

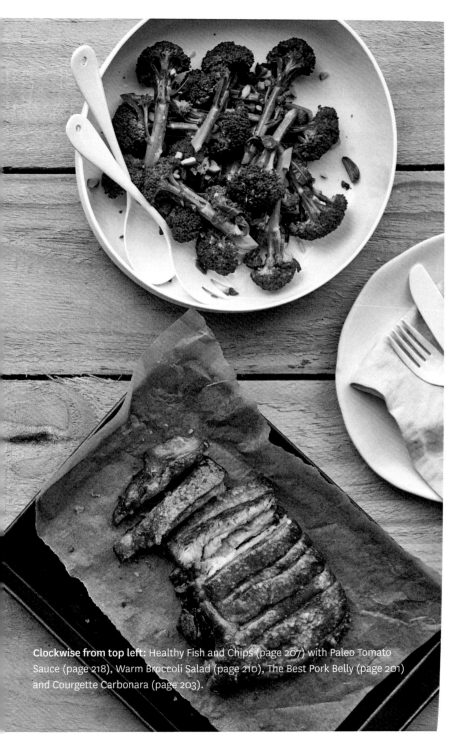

Clockwise from top left: Healthy Fish and Chips (page 207) with Paleo Tomato Sauce (page 218), Warm Broccoli Salad (page 210), The Best Pork Belly (page 201) and Courgette Carbonara (page 203).

SNACKS AND TREATS

Top to bottom: Protein Energy Balls (page 219) and Baked Nut Bars (page 220).

paleo-style diet to operate at its best.

Everyone's nutritional needs are different, and they will also vary according to the type of exercise you are doing. If you are exercising vigorously every day — doing weights at the gym, or running — your nutritional requirements will probably be slightly greater than someone who is doing only light exercise like walking. Your metabolism (the speed at which you break down what you've eaten into products your body can use, such as glycogen and fatty acids for energy or amino acids to repair body tissues or perform bodily functions) varies according to your age and basic genetic make-up, but also significantly according to how much muscle mass you have. So, ironically, an overweight person, who has a larger body mass overall and therefore generally a larger muscle mass (to carry their body weight), can have a higher resting metabolic rate than a slim person. If you are exercising regularly, and therefore increasing your muscle mass, your metabolism will be increasing and therefore your nutritional demands will be increased.

However, the thing is, unless you are an Olympic athlete or an extreme multisporter, or you are seriously into weights and trying to build bulk, you don't need *that much* extra food. And, if one of your goals is to lose weight, you probably don't need any extra food at all.

The big thing an exercising body needs is protein. The body uses carbohydrate for energy, but it gets most of this from glycogen stored in the muscles, not what you eat before a workout. What it needs protein for is

WHAT I ACTUALLY EAT

~ℓℓℓℓ~

You might be wondering how much I actually eat in a day. Surely I must be packing it away if I'm exercising daily? And what am I eating to make up for not consuming grain-based carbohydrates?

Well, you might be surprised. I probably eat less than you think I do — because I eat only what my body needs. So, in an average day, this would be what I would eat.

Breakfast: usually nothing, unless I exercise, in which case I have a protein smoothie.

Lunch: a big, leafy green salad with a sliced chicken breast and a handful of nuts.

Dinner: a single portion of steak (maybe 150 grams uncooked) plus a plateful of veges like broccoli and spinach, or a salad.

Snacks: two black coffees and a green smoothie.

And that is literally all! My body just doesn't need any more food than that for me to work all day and exercise at a high level of intensity.

muscle building and repair. That's why bodybuilders swill down protein powder like it's liquid gold. And if you are doing mostly aerobic or cardiovascular exercise, like gym classes, running or cycling, you are not encouraging a lot of muscle growth, so you don't really need that much extra protein. If you're doing a lot of weight training and you do want to bulk up, you will need to eat more protein so your body has plenty of material to repair damaged muscles and build new ones.

But what about carbs? You need to eat more carbs if you're exercising, to give you energy, right? Wrong again. Unless you are an extreme athlete with a sophisticated regime of carbohydrate depletion and loading before a big event like a marathon, you don't need to eat extra carbs before exercising. You certainly don't need to worry that removing starchy carbs like rice and pasta from your diet is going to affect your exercise performance. Trust me — I exercise every day, either at the gym or playing sport, and I don't ever feel the need to consume those traditional carbs. I thought that I would, based on everything that I had been taught, but that proved to be a myth for me. Eating plenty of vegetables and some fruit gives me all the carbohydrate I need.

PRE-EXERCISE NUTRITION

So, do you need to eat anything special before exercising? This is purely a personal preference and something that you will only figure out by trialling yourself. I used to think you had to eat before working out, even if it was just a banana or a sports drink, but now I usually exercise on an empty stomach and find that works fine for me.

AEROBIC VS ANAEROBIC: HOW YOUR BODY BURNS ENERGY

ℓℓℓℓ

When you're exercising, your body gets the energy it needs from two different places: glycogen (the broken-down form of carbohydrates) stored in your muscles and liver, and stored fat. If you exercise at a low intensity, like walking or swimming, your body is operating in aerobic metabolism mode, using oxygen to burn fat as fuel. If you are doing bursts of high-intensity exercise, like sprints or lifting weights, your body burns glycogen for energy using anaerobic metabolism, and this requires no oxygen.

Your body is very skilled at running the two systems in tandem, and at switching between the two systems. For example, if you are going for a walk your body is getting about 80 per cent of its energy from fat and 20 per cent from glycogen, but if you break into a jog it will change the ratio to about 50:50. If you suddenly do a sprint, it will move to 20:80 in favour of glycogen.

My favourite time to exercise is first thing in the morning, so I usually just get up and go. I admit, this is partly due to the time of day that I exercise — the fitness classes I go to start at 6am, so if I was going to eat first I would have to get up at around 5am, and I don't like the idea of that! I know that when I get up in the morning all the goodness of the nutrition I ate the night before is still in my body, waiting to be used. Your body has huge stores in the liver and muscles of glycogen to provide energy all the time. I don't experience low blood sugar or feel light-headed and am able to exercise at a high level of intensity without eating first in the morning. For me that's just how I operate best.

But everyone's different, so if you feel you do need something a little extra then by all means eat a banana, or something similar — but make sure it's at least an hour before you work out or play sport. It'll take that long to be digested and for the carbohydrate to get into your bloodstream. And you need to have digested whatever you've eaten before you start exercising, because once you are working out, your digestive system effectively switches off — your body diverts blood away from your stomach and intestines and sends it to your muscles. (Check it out: if you touch your tummy while exercising, it will feel quite cold.) It's an evolutionary response, your body's way of putting all its resources into getting you away from danger — running away from sabretooth tigers and the like is when our ancestors used to engage in what we now call physical exercise.

POST-EXERCISE NUTRITION

After exercise, it's a different story. It's very important to replenish your energy stores following an exercise session, and the type and intensity of exercise determines what foods you should consume. You need to put back in what you've taken out of the energy bank — and then a little bit more, so your body can recover and carry out any repairs that need to be done, as well as for muscle growth.

After doing aerobic activity (such as running, cycling or fitness classes) you do need to eat some carbohydrates, in the form of fruit and vegetables, and a lot of water, as you will have lost a lot through sweating and respiration (see the box opposite for some after-exercise snack ideas).

However, if you are doing any exercise, like weight training or the types of exercises in the second section of this book, that gives you sore muscles the next day or the day after, what you need to eat is extra protein so your body can repair torn muscle fibres and build new strong, healthy muscle tissue. That's why and how you develop muscle through weight training: muscle fibre that gets slightly torn through being used and pushed repairs itself slightly bigger, stronger and more resistant to injury. The phrase 'what doesn't kill you makes you stronger' is the human body's motto — when exposed to stressors like exercise it naturally adapts and improves. That sore-muscle feeling is your body's way of telling you to rest so the muscles can repair themselves. If weight training is your thing, you definitely need to increase your protein intake after exercise.

There is a school of thought that says you absorb protein more quickly and efficiently if you eat it at the same time as some carbohydrate, which is why I'll sometimes add a banana to a protein shake following a workout. However, I don't think this is actually a necessity unless you're a serious body-builder type.

You also might hear people talking about the 'protein window' or 'nutrient window', which means if you eat protein within 45 minutes of exercising you'll get the maximum benefit from the amino acids it contains, in terms of rebuilding and growing your muscles. The theory is that the enzymes and hormones in your body responsible for breaking down and absorbing the protein are elevated straight after exercise, so you will absorb the protein more efficiently. I used to think this was really important and tried to follow it religiously, but I have also read other studies which debunk this theory, so I personally don't worry about trying to do this any more. Most of the time I do eat pretty soon after exercising, but this is because I get hungry and I'm all about listening to my body.

AFTER-EXERCISE SNACK IDEAS

On the go: bananas, a can of tuna, hard-boiled eggs, a pre-made protein smoothie (see pages 179–184) or nuts.

In the kitchen: Paleo Pancakes (see page 189) or an Easy Omelette (see page 186).

11. SUPPLEMENTS
THE GOOD, THE BAD
AND THE PROTEIN

• • • • • • • • • • • • • • • •

If you are eating a well-balanced paleo diet, following the guidelines in this book, you should be receiving all the vitamins, minerals and nutrients you need from your mix of healthy carbohydrates, meat, fish, nuts, seeds and, of course, vegetables and fruit. However, you might feel like you want to supplement your diet to increase the amount of certain nutrients you are consuming.

There are two main groups of supplements: everyday supplements, and supplements related to exercise. Here's my list of what's good and useful, and what you just don't need to buy into.

MULTIVITAMINS

I take a multivitamin every day. 'Why?' you might ask. 'Surely you are eating so much good stuff you don't need it?' Well, I just think it's better to be safe than sorry. If you pop a good-quality multivitamin every day, you know you've got your bases covered. It will have all the vitamins your body needs, so if you have a period of time where you aren't eating a specific food, or you can't get a good range of seasonal fruit and veges, you know you are still getting some vital minerals and vitamins. A multivitamin will supplement your diet and keep your body functioning as best it can.

FISH OIL

Fish oils contain omega-3 fatty acids, which are good for your joints, your brain and your skin. There is enough research out there that I am confident that supplementing your diet with fish oil is beneficial and will be better for you long term. Just make sure you are taking a good-quality one: a study in 2015 showed many of the fish oils for sale in New Zealand had lower levels of omega-3s than was claimed on the label. Always make sure you purchase oil from sustainably sourced fish. And remember to keep it in the fridge, or in a dark place, so the oil doesn't start to break down and go rancid.

SUPERFOOD POWDER

I include green superfood powder in my diet every

day, usually added to a Green Smoothie (see page 184). Superfood powder is nutrient dense and is made from things like wheatgrass, spirulina, spinach, flaxseed powder and other vegetable powders. In fact, most green superfood powders contain upwards of 50 different fruits, vegetables and plant foods! Superfood powder contains so many different micronutrients that you probably couldn't get them from your food even if you tried.

I personally feel it gives me energy and makes me feel healthy. Whether or not that is a placebo effect I don't know, but it works for me so, hey, why not? Your brain controls all the processes in your body, so if your brain thinks something is working then it will send out different hormones and change your body chemistry anyway (that's what the placebo effect is).

I usually blend superfood powder up into a smoothie with some kale, kiwifruit and a banana, avocado and water, but you can also take it as a tablet. I like to take as few pills as possible, so the smoothie route works for me.

Read the label and try to choose an organic powder without any extra additives like sweeteners or thickeners.

VITAMIN C (ASCORBIC ACID)

This is one of the key vitamins in terms of maintaining the body's biological processes. It is especially important in helping the body's tissues repair themselves — look what happened to all those old-time scurvy sailors who didn't get enough of it. It also helps your body absorb iron efficiently. Most people take it when they're sick, or when trying to ward off winter colds, but I think it's a good supplement to take all the time, unless you are eating a large amount of vitamin C-rich fruit and vegetables in which case you may not need to take it every day.

The human body can't make its own vitamin C, as most other animals do, so you have to ingest it through food or in a supplement. Vitamin C also can't be stored by the body, so you need to take it regularly. And you can't really overdose on it, as your body will usually just excrete the excess.

SUPPLEMENTS FOR EXERCISE

PROTEIN POWDER

This is the main supplement taken by people who are seriously into exercise. If you are not working out at a high level of intensity on a regular basis, it's a short story: you don't need to be using it as you will be able to get all the protein you need from the food you eat. However, if you are working out at a high intensity, looking to build muscle or are just interested in supplementing your diet with protein powder, here is the low-down.

There are a huge number of different brands and types of protein powder on the market. On my fitness and nutrition journey, I've basically tried everything! I used to try a different one every time I went to the supplements shop. I wanted to find out if any particular type was better for me, producing better results in terms of recovery from training and building muscle.

However, what I found was that they were all pretty similar in terms of providing protein to fuel my muscle recovery. Some of them tasted better and had a more pleasant texture than others, but other than that they seemed to have the same effect.

Then I started to look at the ingredients — where the protein in the powder was coming from (the source), and the other terrible stuff that was being added to them. This really made me rethink consuming this stuff, and I started to look for some more natural options.

There are three main sources of protein in most commercial protein powders: whey (a byproduct of milk production), rice and pea. Like almost everyone I began by using whey protein powders and did so on and off for a number of years. I tried a wide variety of them and found them all very similar.

But as I began to conciously think about what I was putting in my body I also began looking at the ingredients of the powders a little more closely. That is when I became shocked by what was in most of them — artificial sweeteners, sugar, artificial flavourings, preservatives and a whole lot of other chemicals were added to make it act like a powder and mix well with liquid. Whey protein powders also tended to make me (as they do others) bloated and gassy, and hence I was less likely to be invited on long car rides. Anyway, no matter what else is in it, it's still a dairy derivative, so whey protein is out if you are following a paleo lifestyle.

After deciding that my body would be better off without whey protein I started experimenting with pea and rice proteins. I group these two together because they are both very similar in my eyes. The good thing about pea and rice proteins is that a lot of them are far more natural and naturally flavoured than whey proteins. The bad thing about them is that the protein from peas and rice isn't that great for you.

Firstly, peas are legumes and rice is a grain. As we discussed earlier, these foods can contain substances that can cause inflammation in your gut (see page 98 for more on this). Secondly, the protein doesn't have a very good BV (biological value — more on this on page 175), meaning that a lot of the protein doesn't actually get absorbed by your body and instead just passes through you — it's an expensive waste, essentially. And, finally, the texture of these proteins is very chalky, which I didn't like.

The next protein powder I tried and the one I still use every day is the CleanPaleo protein powder that we make. Our protein powders are made from free-range egg white and flavoured with natural wholefood ingredients. They don't contain dairy, refined sugar, preservatives or anything artificial. I honestly believe that these powders are the best protein powders for the human body. Egg protein is an extremely high-quality protein, rich in the branched-chain amino acids (BCAAs) that help to promote protein and muscle synthesis in the body. I think having a powder like this is the most natural way to conveniently get extra protein into your body without adding any other nasty stuff.

I'm not a bodybuilder, so I don't really need to be using protein powder. However, I use it because of the convenience: if I have a smoothie with added protein powder for breakfast, I can take in the same amount of protein as if I ate four eggs or a cooked breakfast — but I can do it in the car on the way to work! It's a lot easier to make a smoothie and rinse out the blender than to whip up an omelette and have to wash the bowl, the frying pan and the plate, too! Protein helps you to feel full for longer, so a protein smoothie in the morning sets you up really well for the day.

The other advantage is that because you are consuming the protein in a powder form, in a drink, it is more easily absorbed by the body, with less stress on your digestive system. It helps your body to repair itself after exercise and replenish the glycogen stores in your muscles and liver.

Basically, what I look for in protein powder is something that sits well with my body, isn't going to negatively affect it in any way, and is going to give me the greatest possible benefit.

BAD SUPPLEMENTS

So, what should you avoid using? In my opinion, any pre-workout supplements are bad news. They are usually just full of chemicals and have drug-like effects on your brain and your body. They are so artificial it's

BV (BIOLOGICAL VALUE)

All proteins — and therefore all protein powders — have a biological value or BV, which is is a measure (between 0 and 100) of how efficiently a protein is metabolised, absorbed and used by your body. Eggs are considered by nutritionists as one of the most bioavailable sources of protein, which is why the biological value (BV) scale is based on egg protein: egg gets a BV value of 100 and sets the scale.

Unlike fat and carbohydrate, which can be stored by the body, any excess protein not used by the body is excreted, so it makes sense to consume proteins with a high BV, to get the best bang for your buck.

The natural protein powder with the highest BV — that is, the most absorbable protein — is egg, which has a BV of 100. Whey protein historically was around 90 per cent, however, some new-generation, highly 'micronised' (very fine) whey protein powders have a BV of more than 100. Rice protein powders have a BV of about 76; and pea protein powders bring up the rear with a BV of around 65.

If you want to get the most out of the protein you are consuming, this is another reason to go for egg protein powder. Or, better still, just eat the real thing!

frightening. They taste like supercharged, jacked-up, hyper-sweet fruit that punch you in the taste buds and make your face tingle (at least that's what they did to me). They have no place in a paleo lifestyle or any lifestyle for anyone who cares about their body.

And then there's fat-burning supplements, or thermogenics. Thermogenic means 'to produce heat', and these drugs basically cause an increase in your body temperature through metabolic stimulation. They increase your basal metabolic rate (resting metabolism), causing you to increase your energy expenditure. They are incredibly unnatural and affect your body in a very artificial and sometimes dangerous way. They are very bad for you and I urge everyone to stay away from them.

However, if you are absolutely dead set on taking something to give you increased energy and focus for your workout, you can get pretty much the same effect as these expensive supplements by having a coffee. Yes, a coffee. Caffeine is one of the key ingredients in most of these pre-workout supplements, because it makes you feel like you've got more energy since it tells your brain to produce adrenalin, which is a stress hormone.

Plus, most of these supplements are just marketing nonsense: they're not going to make a difference to your workout if you are just an average guy or girl. So much so-called 'sports nutrition' is just dodgy marketing, cashing in on the fact that everyone wants to be like the All Blacks or their other sporting heroes. They want to be lean, muscular and fit while expending the least amount of energy possible. And that's where supplement marketers take advantage of people — by promising a shortcut to amazing results. But the price you pay is your long-term health. Turn your back on them and you'll feel much better, I promise.

12. PALEO RECIPES

ℓℓℓℓ

In the following pages you will find some of my favourite go-to paleo recipes. Some of the ingredients might not be available in supermarkets. but you should be able to find them at good health-food shops. online or from CleanPaleo. Enjoy!

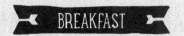
⊱SMOOTHIES⊰

In the following smoothie recipes. adding protein powder is optional. If you are going to have just a smoothie for breakfast. or are planning to exercise. then the protein powder will help you to get through the morning without needing to snack. However. you don't have to add the protein powder if you're having a smoothie as a snack or with another breakfast food.

SALTED CARAMEL SMOOTHIE

— SERVES 1 —

1 cup almond milk

1 cup coconut milk

1 ripe banana

1 Medjool date, pitted

2 tablespoons CleanPaleo Native Vanilla Protein (optional)

2 teaspoons maple syrup

½ teaspoon sea salt

handful of ice

1 free-range egg (optional)

Place all ingredients in a blender, and blend to combine.

VANILLA, BANANA AND COCONUT SMOOTHIE

1½ cups coconut milk
1 ripe banana
1 Medjool date, pitted
2 tablespoons CleanPaleo Native Vanilla Protein (optional)
1 teaspoon ground cinnamon
handful of ice
chopped raw almonds, to serve (optional)
unsweetened shredded coconut, to serve (optional)

Place all ingredients in a blender, and blend to combine.
Serve topped with chopped raw almonds and unsweetened
shredded coconut, if you wish.

BERRY SMOOTHIE

1 cup almond milk
½ cup coconut milk
1 ripe banana, peeled
1 medjool date, pitted
1 ½ handfuls of fresh or frozen berries of your choice
1 handful of ice

Place all ingredients in a blender and combine. Serve topped
with fresh berries if you wish.

CHOCOLATE SMOOTHIE

2 cups almond milk

1 ripe banana

1 Medjool date, pitted

2 tablespoons CleanPaleo Native Vanilla Protein (optional)

3 tablespoons raw cacao powder

1 teaspoon raw honey or maple syrup

handful of ice

1 free-range egg (optional)

unsweetened shredded coconut, to serve (optional)

Place all ingredients in a blender, and blend to combine. Serve topped with unsweetened shredded coconut, if you wish.

MOCHACCINO
WAKE-UP SMOOTHIE

— SERVES 1 —

1 cup almond milk

1 cup coconut milk

1 ripe banana

1 Medjool date, pitted

2 tablespoons CleanPaleo Mochaccino Protein, or 1 shot of espresso

2 teaspoons maple syrup

handful of ice

Place all ingredients in a blender, and blend to combine.

GREEN SMOOTHIE

This is one of my favourite easy breakfasts.

— SERVES 1 —

1 cup water
1 ripe banana
1 green kiwifruit, peeled
handful of kale leaves, stems discarded
½ avocado, halved, stone removed and peeled
1 tablespoon superfood powder
handful of ice
chopped kiwifruit, to serve (optional)
fresh mint sprigs, to serve (optional)

Place all ingredients in a blender, and blend to combine. Serve topped with chopped kiwifruit and fresh mint, if you wish.

WELLNESS JUICE

This is a great pick-me-up full of vitamins.
Perfect if you are feeling a bit under the weather.
or to make for a friend who is sick. You'll need a juicer.
Another good addition is 1 tablespoon lemon juice.

— **MAKES ENOUGH FOR 2 PEOPLE** —

3 medium-sized beetroot, trimmed, peeled and cut into pieces

2 large carrots, peeled and cut into pieces

1 large apple, peeled and cut into pieces

2.5cm piece fresh ginger (or more to taste),
peeled and cut into pieces

1 large orange or grapefruit, peeled

Juice everything in a juicer, then stir to combine. Serve in
two glasses.

EASY OMELETTE

Omelettes are really easy to make and are totally paleo — they are just eggs and a little water with whatever filling you choose. You can also include cheese if you like (I do!). Coconut oil has a slightly nutty taste, so use olive oil if you prefer.

— **MAKES 1 OMELETTE** —

2–3 free-range eggs

2 tablespoons water

salt and freshly ground black pepper, to taste

1 tablespoon coconut oil or olive oil, for cooking

suggested fillings: chopped ham; chopped, lightly cooked bacon; chopped, cooked chicken; chopped red capsicum; chopped tomato; chopped red onion; chopped avocado; handful of grated Gruyère cheese

chopped flat-leaf parsley, to serve (optional)

Place the eggs in a bowl and lightly beat with a fork. Add the water and season with salt and pepper.

Melt the coconut oil or heat the olive oil in a small frying pan, and season well with salt and pepper. When hot, tip in the egg and tilt the pan so that the egg covers the base. Using a spatula, drag the cooked egg to the centre, allowing the uncooked egg to flow to the edges. Repeat this once more.

Spoon over your chosen fillings and fold the furthest part of the omelette over top of the filling. As a rough guide, use about 1½ handfuls total of filling so that you don't overfill your omlette.

Slide the cooked omelette on to a warm plate, garnish with parsley and eat.

EGGS BENEDICT WITH PALEO HOLLANDAISE

This is a classic breakfast dish. Of course, this version doesn't have the bread or the English muffin underneath the egg. Try it on a Kumara Rosti (see page 213), or you can lay it on a bed of ham, cooked bacon, wilted spinach, steamed asparagus or cooked salmon (or a combination of these!), then smother it with delicious paleo hollandaise.

Use coconut oil or clarified butter for the hollandaise, depending on your preference and to what extent you're avoiding dairy.

— MAKES ENOUGH FOR 2–3 PEOPLE —

PALEO HOLLANDAISE

3 free-range egg yolks

1 tablespoon lemon juice

½ teaspoon sea salt

½ cup hot, melted clarified butter,
or ¼ cup hot, melted coconut oil

Place the egg yolks, lemon juice and sea salt in a blender, and blend until combined. Slowly pour in the very hot butter or oil until the mixture thickens.

Set aside in a warm place while you poach the eggs.

Recipe continued over the page . . .

POACHED EGGS

1–2 free-range eggs per person
your choice of base
smoked paprika, to serve

Fill a deep frying pan or wide saucepan with at least 10cm of lightly salted water, and bring to a simmer.

Break each egg into a cup to ensure the yolk stays intact. Stir the water in the pan with a spoon to create a whirlpool, then drop each egg into the centre and wait for 3–4 minutes — you can poach up to four eggs at a time. Remove the eggs with a slotted spoon, drain on a folded paper towel, then slide on to your preferred base combination.

Spoon a little hollandaise over each egg and sprinkle with smoked paprika.

PALEO PANCAKES

Add some protein powder to this pancake mixture
before frying for extra sustenance.

— MAKES ABOUT 24 SMALL PANCAKES —

4 free-range eggs
2 ripe bananas, lightly mashed
1 teaspoon baking powder
coconut oil, to cook
fresh berries, to serve
maple syrup, to serve
coconut whip, to serve (optional)

Place the eggs, banana and baking powder in a blender or food
processor, and blend until thick.

Heat a little coconut oil in a non-stick frying pan over a
medium-low heat. Drop in dessertspoonfuls of the pancake
mixture, and cook until golden, then turn over and cook the
other side until also golden. Repeat with the remaining mixture.

Place the pancakes on a warm plate as you go, and cover them
with a clean tea towel.

Serve your pancakes topped with sliced or whole fresh berries
and drizzle with maple syrup and a dollop of coconut whip, if
you wish. (To make coconut whip, simply whip a can of chilled
coconut cream.)

PALEO NUT AND SEED BREAD

If you really can't live without a toast substitute at breakfast, try this amazing paleo bread. This recipe is a slight variation on My New Roots' Life-changing Loaf of Bread, and they don't call it life-changing for nothing! The original recipe can be found online at mynewroots.org

— MAKES 1 LOAF —

1½ cups wholegrain rolled oats (not quick-cook oats)

1 cup sunflower seeds

½ cup raw almonds

½ cup flaxseed

¼ cup psyllium seed husks

2 tablespoons chia seeds

1 teaspoon sea salt

1½ cups cold water

3 tablespoons melted coconut oil

1 tablespoon maple syrup

Line a large loaf tin (about 20cm x 14cm x 7cm deep) with baking paper.

In a large bowl, combine all of the dry ingredients.

In another bowl, whisk together the water, coconut oil and maple syrup.

Add the wet ingredients to the dry ingredients, and mix well until the dough is very thick. Spoon it into the prepared loaf tin, then cover and leave to stand in a cool place in your kitchen for at least 2 hours, but preferably all day or overnight.

Preheat the oven to 175°C.

Place the loaf on the middle rack in the oven and bake for 20 minutes. Remove from the oven, and take the loaf out of the tin. Place it upside down directly on the oven rack and continue to bake for another 30–40 minutes — it is cooked when it sounds hollow when tapped on the base.

Remove from the oven and allow to cool completely on a wire rack before slicing.

Store in an airtight container at room temperature for up to four days, or freeze.

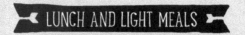
BEETROOT AND CARROT SALAD

Add a meat of your choice if you want
to increase your protein intake.

— SERVES 4 —

2 large carrots, scrubbed
2 medium-sized beetroot, peeled
handful of sultanas
juice of 1 lemon

Coarsely grate the carrots and beetroot, and place in a large
bowl. Add the sultanas and lemon juice, and stir gently to
combine.

SPINACH, BASIL AND BACON FRITTATA

A green salad is a great accompaniment for this frittata.

— SERVES 4 —

4 rashers rindless bacon, chopped
8 free-range eggs, at room temperature
2 tablespoons almond milk
¼ cup small basil leaves
salt and freshly ground black pepper, to taste
1 tablespoon olive oil
4 handfuls of baby spinach leaves
1 large, ripe tomato, sliced and seeds removed
chopped flat-leaf parsley, to garnish (optional)

Preheat the oven to 180°C.

Place the chopped bacon in a 24cm frying pan that can also go in the oven, and cook over a medium heat until it just begins to colour. Transfer it to a plate and set aside.

In a bowl, whisk together the eggs, almond milk and basil leaves. Season with salt and freshly ground black pepper.

Add the olive oil to the frying pan and heat to a medium heat, then add the baby spinach and cook until wilted. Return the bacon to the pan, and stir to combine.

Pour in the egg mixture and place the tomato slices on top. Allow the frittata to set on the base, then transfer it to the oven and cook until the top is just set and beginning to colour, but be careful not to overcook it. Remove from the oven and cut into wedges to serve. Garnish with parsley if you wish.

CHICKEN AND AVOCADO SALAD

As a variation to this recipe, you could barbecue the chicken breasts — but leave the skin on to protect the meat and add flavour. You might also scatter over some fresh summer herbs, such as basil, dill, sweet marjoram or chives.

— SERVES 4 —

3–4 skinless free-range chicken breasts

2 cups hot chicken stock

2 tablespoons olive oil

juice of 1 lemon

4 large handfuls of mesclun — you can also use baby cos or shredded iceberg lettuce

1 large, ripe but firm avocado, halved, stone removed, peeled and sliced

1 red capsicum, deseeded and thinly sliced

extra lemon juice and olive oil, to serve

salt and freshly ground black pepper, to taste

Place the chicken breasts in a large, wide saucepan, and cover with the hot stock. Place over the heat, bring the stock back up to the boil, then reduce the heat and simmer, turning the chicken halfway through, for 8–12 minutes or until the chicken is just cooked. Remove the saucepan from the heat and allow to cool.

Once the chicken is cool, remove it from the stock. You can freeze the stock to use later in another recipe.

Shred the chicken by pulling the meat apart with your hands — pulling the chicken apart like this gives you meat that is ultimately more succulent.

Place the chicken in a bowl with 2 tablespoons olive oil and the juice of 1 lemon.

Place the mesclun on a platter, and top it with the chicken, oil and lemon juice.

Scatter over the avocado and red capsicum slices, then squeeze over the extra lemon juice and drizzle with the extra olive oil. Season with salt and freshly ground black pepper.

PALEO WRAPS MEXICAN-STYLE

Hola! These cos lettuce wraps are a great alternative
to a carbohydrate wrap or sandwich. Use whatever
fillings take your fancy. My favourite combination is
chicken and avocado, but feel free to experiment as I
have done with this Mexican-style version.

— SERVES 4 —

2 x 200g beef steaks

1 teaspoon paprika

¼ teaspoon ground cumin

1 tablespoon olive oil

1 large, ripe avocado

juice of 1 lemon

good pinch of sea salt

12 cos lettuce leaves, to serve

1 red capsicum, deseeded and thinly sliced

1 small red onion, peeled and thinly sliced

1 tablespoon pumpkin seeds,
preferably dry roasted for added flavour

a few coriander leaves

1 red or green chilli, thinly sliced

juice of 2 limes, to serve

Rub the beef steaks with the paprika, ground cumin and oil,
then cook until rare (3–4 minutes on each side in a hot pan).
Rest before cutting into thin slices.

Mash the avocado with the lemon juice and salt to make
guacamole.

Lay the lettuce leaves out on a board and fill each with slices of
beef, then top with guacamole, capsicum, red onion, pumpkin
seeds, coriander and chilli. Squeeze over the lime juice and EAT!

THAI-SCENTED PUMPKIN SOUP

— SERVES 2-3 —

2 teaspoons coconut oil
1 onion, peeled and finely chopped
1 stalk lemongrass, white part only, cut in half
2cm piece fresh ginger, peeled
4 kaffir lime leaves
1 red chilli, deseeded and sliced
1 tablespoon chopped coriander stalks
1 teaspoon ground turmeric
3 cups deseeded, peeled and diced pumpkin
1 litre vegetable or chicken stock
½ cup coconut cream
salt and freshly ground black pepper, to taste
1 tablespoon roughly chopped coriander leaves, to serve
juice of 2-3 limes, to serve

Put the coconut oil in a medium-sized saucepan and place over a medium-low heat. Add the onion, lemongrass, ginger, kaffir lime leaves, chilli and coriander stalks, and cook for 2–3 minutes. Add the turmeric, and cook for a further 30 seconds. Add the pumpkin and stock. Lower the heat and simmer, covered, until the pumpkin is soft.

Remove from the heat and leave to stand for 5 minutes.

Remove the lemongrass, ginger and kaffir lime leaves, and discard. Blend the soup in a blender until smooth then reheat it in the saucepan. Add the coconut cream and season to taste.

To serve, divide the soup between warmed soup bowls, scatter over the coriander leaves and squeeze over plenty of lime juice.

VEGETABLE AND CHICKEN SOUP

Dice the root vegetables so they will easily sit on a soup spoon when eating. The spinach can be replaced with other green vegetables. such as kale or cabbage. but adjust the cooking time accordingly so they are tender before you add the chicken.

— SERVES 4 —

2 tablespoons olive oil

1 onion, peeled and diced

2 cloves garlic, peeled and finely chopped

2 carrots, peeled and diced

2 sticks of celery, stringy bits removed
with a vegetable peeler and diced

1 red kumara, peeled and diced

400g can chopped tomatoes in juice

4 cups vegetable or chicken stock

2 teaspoons chopped fresh sweet marjoram or oregano leaves

2 handfuls of baby spinach leaves

1 cup cooked, diced chicken

salt and freshly ground black pepper, to taste

Put the olive oil in a large saucepan and place over a low heat. Add the onion and cook for about 10 minutes, until the onion is soft and just beginning to colour. Add the garlic, carrots, celery and kumara, and cook for a further 2 minutes, tossing to coat in the onion mixture. Add the tomatoes, stock and sweet marjoram or oregano, and bring to the boil. Lower the heat and simmer for about 20 minutes, until the vegetables are tender.

Add the baby spinach and chicken. Cook for 5 minutes, until the chicken is heated through. Season with salt and pepper.

Serve hot with Paleo Nut and Seed Bread (see page 190).

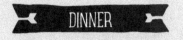

PALEO BURGERS

I really like making paleo burgers by replacing the buns
with lettuce leaves, tomato slices or large, meaty roasted
mushrooms. Who needs that soggy bun, anyway?!

— MAKES 4 BURGERS —

500g beef mince
1 tablespoon chopped fresh parsley
1 teaspoon dried oregano, or your favourite seasoning powder
salt and freshly ground black pepper, to taste
10 small pickling onions, peeled and quartered
¼ cup olive oil
1 bay leaf
good splash of balsamic vinegar
dash of olive oil, to cook
1 large, ripe but firm tomato
1 ripe but firm avocado, halved, stone removed, peeled and sliced
small basil leaves, to serve

Place the beef mince in a bowl and add the parsley and
oregano or seasoning powder, and season with salt and freshly
ground black pepper. Divide the beef mince into four and
shape into patties. Place the patties on a plate, cover and
refrigerate until ready to cook.

Put the onions, oil and bay leaf in a heavy-based saucepan, and
place over a medium-low heat. Cover and cook for 15 minutes,
until the onions begin to soften — shake the pan from time to
time to ensure they are not sticking.

Recipe continued over the page . . .

Remove the lid and continue to cook, stirring until the onions have separated and are turning a rich golden colour and are full of flavour. Remove from the heat and add balsamic vinegar.

Remove the beef patties from the refrigerator and bring to room temperature. Heat a large frying pan over a medium heat and add a dash of olive oil. Add the patties and cook, turning once, for 5–8 minutes on each side, depending on the thickness of your patties.

Cut the tomato into four thick slices and place a patty on top of each slice. Top with the caramelised onion and the avocado slices. Sprinkle with fresh basil leaves and eat. Pass the salt and pepper!

THE BEST PORK BELLY

If you are buying pork belly from your local butcher,
ask them to score the skin for you. Sometimes it
is already scored, but add a few more cuts for even
better results. You will need a roasting dish with
roasting rack. Serve this pork belly with Kumara Mash
(see page 214) and an Asian-style slaw.

— SERVES 6 —

2kg free-range pork belly
olive oil, for rubbing
2 tablespoons fennel seeds, ground
sea salt, to sprinkle

Preheat the oven to 130°C.

Place the pork belly skin side up on the rack of a roasting dish.
Use paper towels to pat the skin dry.

Rub the pork belly on both sides with olive oil, then rub both
sides with the ground fennel. Sprinkle sea salt on the skin side
only and rub it in.

Place the pork belly in the oven and roast for 3 hours (check
after 2 hours to see how it is roasting — you want the meat to
be tender).

Remove from the oven and turn the oven to grill. Grill the pork
belly for about 5 minutes, keeping an eye on it to make sure it
doesn't burn, to get the skin crackling.

CARAMELISED SALMON

This recipe uses coconut aminos. which is made from fermented coconut sap and salt. It can be used as a healthy alternative to soy sauce. Coconut aminos has lots of amino acids and doesn't taste of coconut at all.

— SERVES 4 —

4 salmon fillets (about 150g each), skin on and bones removed
coconut sugar, for rubbing
4 tablespoons coconut aminos

Preheat the oven to 200°C. Line a shallow baking tray with baking paper.

Place the salmon fillets skin side down on the tray. Rub the salmon flesh with coconut sugar and drizzle with the coconut aminos.

Place in the oven and cook for about 10 minutes, or until the salmon flakes away easily and looks caramelised.

⊷PALEO PASTA⊷

Just because you are following a paleo lifestyle doesn't
mean you shouldn't tuck into a plate of 'pasta' from time
to time. The following recipe uses strips of courgette as
the pasta, which doesn't need prior cooking. You can also
make vegetable pasta from strips of carrot. To make your
courgette pasta, use a vegetable peeler or spiraliser and
only use the outer layers, not the weird core part —
I think it tastes a bit average!

COURGETTE CARBONARA
— SERVES 3-4 —

250g streaky bacon, rind removed

250g button mushrooms, halved if large

6 courgettes, ends trimmed off

6 free-range eggs

¾ cup coconut milk

3 cloves garlic, peeled and crushed

1 teaspoon dried basil

1 teaspoon dried oregano

1 teaspoon dried parsley

sea salt, to taste

1 tablespoon finely chopped fresh parsley

freshly grated Parmesan cheese (optional)

freshly ground black pepper, to taste

Heat a large frying pan over a medium-high heat and add the
bacon. Pan-fry until golden and crisp. Remove the bacon and
set aside.

Recipe continued over the page . . .

Add the mushrooms to the pan and cook until browned, then remove and set aside. Set the frying pan aside, but don't wash it.

Peel the courgettes into thick strips using a vegetable peeler, and set aside.

Crack the eggs into a bowl and lightly whisk. Add the coconut milk, garlic and dried herbs, and lightly whisk to combine. Season with sea salt.

Return the frying pan with bacon fat still in it to a medium heat. When hot, pour in the egg mixture. Add the courgette strips and the bacon, and cook until the egg mixture just begins to set around the courgette.

Spoon into a large, warm pasta bowl, sprinkle with the chopped parsley and Parmesan cheese (if using), and serve. Pass the black pepper grinder!

TWO MORE IDEAS

Chicken Pesto Courgette Fettuccine: make a pesto sauce using your favourite pesto, and warm it with crushed garlic and cream. Toss your courgette strips in the sauce, along with cooked chicken and cooked mushrooms.

Chicken and Chorizo Fettucine: make a tomato sauce with olive oil, crushed garlic, 400g can chopped tomatoes in juice, tomato paste and even a splash of red wine for extra flavour. Toss your courgette strips in the tomato sauce with cooked chicken and cooked, sliced chorizo.

AUBERGINE LASAGNE

This is simply a lasagne, just using aubergine instead
of pasta. You can cook the aubergine slices in a frying
pan, grill in the oven or outside on your barbecue.

— SERVES 4 —

1 large aubergine, cut into slices lengthwise

½ cup coconut oil, melted

1 onion, peeled and finely chopped

350g pork mince

350g beef mince

4 cloves garlic, peeled and crushed

400g can chopped tomatoes in juice

¼ cup tomato paste

¼ cup finely chopped fresh parsley

2 tablespoons torn fresh basil leaves

1 tablespoon chopped fresh oregano leaves

1 tablespoon chopped fresh thyme leaves

1 teaspoon fennel seeds

salt and freshly ground black pepper, to taste

2 free-range eggs, beaten

Heat a large frying pan over a medium-high heat. Brush the
aubergine slices liberally with coconut oil. Cook in batches in
the frying pan, until dark golden and tender. Remove from the
pan and set aside.

Heat the remaining coconut oil in the frying pan over a low
heat. Add the onion and cook until soft. Add the pork and beef
mince, turn up the heat and brown the meat, stirring with a
wooden spoon to break it up.

Recipe continued over the page . . .

Add the garlic, chopped tomatoes, tomato paste, fresh herbs and fennel seeds. Lower the heat, cover the frying pan and simmer for 20–30 minutes, stirring from time to time. Season with salt and freshly ground black pepper.

Preheat the oven to 175°C. Grease a medium-sized ovenproof baking dish.

Stir the beaten eggs into the mince mixture. Place half of the meat mixture into the base of the ovenproof dish. Top with half of the aubergine slices. Repeat with the remaining mince mixture and finish with the remaining aubergine slices.

Cover the dish with foil and place in the oven to cook for 20 minutes, until hot and bubbling.

ONE MORE IDEA

You could use chicken mince instead of the beef and pork, and replace the aubergine slices with grilled streaky bacon. Did someone say 'meatsagne'?!

HEALTHY FISH AND CHIPS

— SERVES 4 —

8 small red kumara, skin on
¼ cup coconut oil
4 fish fillets — you can use delicate, medium or firm-fleshed fish
1 cup almond meal
1 tablespoon coconut oil
lemon wedges, to serve
Paleo Tomato Sauce, to serve (see page 218)

Preheat the oven to 200°C.

Boil the whole kumara in lightly salted water until just tender. Drain and cut into wedges.

Meanwhile, heat ¼ cup coconut oil in a shallow roasting dish. When hot, add the kumara wedges and toss to coat them in the oil. Spread the wedges into a single layer and return the roasting dish to the oven. Roast the kumara for 15–20 minutes, until golden and crisp.

Coat the fish fillets in the almond meal. Heat 1 tablespoon coconut oil in a large frying pan over a medium heat and add the fish. Cook for a few minutes on each side, until golden — the cooking time will depend on the thickness of the fillets.

Serve your fish and chips with lemon wedges for squeezing and some Paleo Tomato Sauce on the side, of course.

MEATZA

The ultimate pizza for meat lovers! Think pizza with mince forming the crust rather than the traditional bread dough. When I made this for my flatmates. we tried to put as many different kinds of meat on top as we could. but you can keep it reasonable and just go for a vegetable combo as in the recipe below.

— SERVES 3-4 —

750g–1kg beef mince
1 onion, peeled and very finely chopped
1 clove garlic, peeled and crushed
1 free-range egg
½ cup freshly grated Parmesan cheese (optional)
salt and freshly ground black pepper, to taste
¼ cup tomato paste
400g can Roma tomatoes, drained
1 tablespoon olive oil
½ green capsicum, deseeded and sliced
½ red capsicum, deseeded and sliced
4 spring onions, finely sliced
¼ cup fresh basil leaves
2 tablespoons fresh sweet marjoram or oregano leaves
250–300g buffalo mozzarella, torn into pieces (optional)

Preheat the oven to 220°C. Line a large, shallow baking tray with baking paper.

In a large bowl, mix together the beef mince, onion, garlic, egg and Parmesan cheese (if using), and season well with salt and freshly ground black pepper.

Place the meat on the prepared tray and, using wet hands, flatten it out as thinly as possible. Cover with cling film and use a rolling pin to roll it even thinner. Remove the cling film.

Place the meat in the oven. Cook for 10 minutes then remove from the oven and reduce the oven temperature to 175°C.

Spread the tomato paste over the meat.

Roughly chop the canned tomatoes and mix with the olive oil, then season and spread over the tomato paste.

Top with the capsicum slices, spring onion and fresh herbs.

Scatter over the pieces of buffalo mozzarella (if using) and return to the oven to cook for a further 10 minutes, until the cheese has melted. Pass the pepper grinder, and bring on the meat sweats!

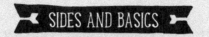

WARM BROCCOLI SALAD

— SERVES 4 AS A SIDE DISH —

1 large head broccoli
2 tablespoons olive oil
3 cloves garlic, peeled and sliced
1 red chilli, deseeded and finely sliced
salt and freshly ground black pepper, to taste
good handful of raw almonds, roughly chopped
1 lemon, to serve

Cut the broccoli into florets and steam until tender.

Heat the oil in a frying pan, and pan-fry the garlic and chilli for 30 seconds on a medium heat, ensuring they do not burn. Add the broccoli and cook until hot.

Place in a big serving bowl, and season with salt and freshly ground black pepper. Scatter over the almonds and squeeze over the lemon juice.

BOK CHOY STIR-FRY

Asian greens are perfect for stir-frying —
they love it hot and steamy. You can add meat
or fish to this dish as well.

— SERVES 4 AS A SIDE DISH —

4 whole baby bok choy
1 tablespoon olive oil or coconut oil
1 tablespoon peeled and finely shredded fresh ginger
1 clove garlic, peeled and crushed
1 tablespoon coconut aminos

Steam the baby bok choy for about 1 minute.

Heat the oil in a wok, and stir-fry the ginger and garlic. Add the steamed baby bok choy, and toss to coat. When hot, stir in the coconut aminos.

Pile in a serving dish and serve hot.

CAULIFLOWER COUSCOUS

Cauliflower couscous can also be eaten raw. Use it
as you would couscous, mixed with lots of fresh
herbs and drizzled with plenty of lemon juice.

— **SERVES 3-4** —

½ head cauliflower
1 tablespoon olive oil
sea salt, to taste

Cut the cauliflower into florets. Trim the stalks and refrigerate for
another use — for example, they would be great in a stir-fry.

Place the cauliflower florets in a food processor and, in two
separate batches to prevent overcrowding the processor,
process until the cauliflower resembles couscous.

Heat the olive oil in a large frying pan over a medium heat.
Add the cauliflower couscous and season with sea salt.
Cover and cook for about 5 minutes, until tender.

KUMARA ROSTI

I recommend orange kumara for this recipe. as the flesh
is softer in texture and therefore cooks more easily.
These rosti make a great English-muffin alternative
to go with Paleo Eggs Benedict (see page 187).

— SERVES 4 —

4 cups peeled, coarsely grated orange kumara
4 spring onions, finely chopped
1 tablespoon finely chopped fresh parsley or dill
1 teaspoon chopped thyme leaves
1 free-range egg
salt and freshly ground black pepper, to taste
1 tablespoon coconut oil

Preheat the oven to 180°C. Line a shallow baking tray with
baking paper.

Squeeze as much liquid as you can from the grated kumara,
then place it in a bowl with the spring onion, fresh herbs and
egg. Mix well, and season with salt and freshly ground black
pepper.

Melt the coconut oil in a large frying pan over a medium heat.
Drop four large spoonfuls of the rosti mixture into the frying
pan and flatten each with a spatula — press down hard to
press mixture together. Cook until golden, then carefully flip
over and cook on the other side until also golden. Transfer to
the baking tray. Repeat with the remaining mixture.

Place the rosti in the oven and cook for 15 minutes until tender.

KUMARA MASH

— SERVES 2 —

2 red kumara, peeled and cut into chunks
15g butter
¼ cup almond milk or coconut milk, warmed
salt and freshly ground black pepper, to taste

Boil the kumara in lightly salted water until tender. Drain and dry off in the pan over the heat.

Mash the kumara, then beat in the butter and warmed milk. Season with salt and freshly ground black pepper.

ALMOND MILK

1 cup raw almonds
3 cups water
pinch of sea salt

Place the almonds in a bowl and just cover with cold water. Leave to soak in a cool place overnight. Drain, discard the liquid and rinse.

Place the soaked almonds in a blender and add 3 cups water and sea salt. Blend until smooth.

Line a large sieve with cheesecloth, then place it over a jug. Pour the almond milk from the blender into the lined sieve. Finish by squeezing the cheesecloth to extract all of the almond milk.

Keep in the refrigerator for up to four days.

PROPER ALMOND BUTTER

Soaking the nuts makes them easier to
digest and improves the flavour.

— MAKES 1 CUP —

2 cups raw almonds
1 tablespoon coconut oil
sea salt, to taste

Place the almonds in a bowl and cover with cold water. Leave
in a cool place to soak for 8 hours. Drain, discard the liquid
and rinse.

Preheat the oven to a very low temperature, about 100°C.

Spread the nuts out in a single layer on a baking tray and place
in the oven. Leave the nuts in the oven until completely dry and
crisp — this can take 12 hours or more.

Now that the almonds have been soaked and dehydrated,
place them in a food processor and process to a fine powder.
Add the coconut oil and continue to process until smooth and
creamy — this may take a while. Add sea salt to taste.

PALEO MAYONNAISE

Ensure that all your ingredients are at room
temperature before you begin. You can add an extra
egg white or some extra lemon juice if you
want a thinner mayonnaise.

— MAKES ABOUT 1 CUP —

3 free-range egg yolks
1 teaspoon Dijon mustard
250ml olive oil
sea salt, to taste
lemon juice, to taste

Place the egg yolks and mustard in the bowl of a small food
processor. Process until combined, then very slowly drizzle in
the olive oil. Season with sea salt and lemon juice.

Spoon into a bowl or jar, cover well and place in the refrigerator
for up to one week.

PALEO TOMATO SAUCE

— MAKES ABOUT 1 CUP —

⅔ cup tomato paste
2 tablespoons cider vinegar
¼ teaspoon mustard powder
¼ teaspoon cinnamon
¼ teaspoon sea salt
good pinch of ground allspice
⅓ cup cold water

Place all ingredients except for the water in a bowl, then whisk in the cold water — add more water if needed to thin the sauce.

Refrigerate overnight to allow flavours to mingle before using. Keep in the refrigerator for up to one week.

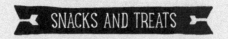

PROTEIN ENERGY BALLS

— MAKES 24 BALLS —

10 Medjool dates, pitted
½ cup macadamia nuts
½ cup raw almonds
½ cup CleanPaleo Native Vanilla Protein
3 tablespoons raw cacao powder
4 tablespoons coconut butter
1 tablespoon raw honey or maple syrup
2 teaspoons vanilla powder, such as Heilala Vanilla Powder
pinch of sea salt
¼ cup raw cacao powder, to coat

Place all ingredients except for the second measure of raw cacao powder in a food processor, and process until sticky.

Take rounded teaspoonfuls of the mixture and roll into 24 balls, then roll to coat in the raw cacao powder.

Store in an airtight container in the refrigerator for up to one week.

BAKED NUT BARS

— MAKES ABOUT 12 BARS —

1 cup raw cashew nuts

½ cup raw almonds

½ cup pecans

½ cup unsweetened shredded coconut

zest of 1 small orange

½ cup raw honey

1 teaspoon vanilla extract

½ teaspoon sea salt

Preheat the oven to 175°C. Line a 20cm x 20cm square cake tin with baking paper.

Roughly chop the nuts by hand, then place them in a large bowl with the remaining ingredients. Mix well.

Spoon into the cake tin and bake in the oven for 20 minutes.

Remove from the oven and allow to cool completely before cutting into bars.

Store in an airtight container at room temperature, layering with baking paper to prevent the bars from sticking together, for up to four days.

MEDJOOL DATE
RAW ENERGY BARS

— MAKES ABOUT 24 SMALL BARS —

10 Medjool dates, pitted
1 cup raw cashew nuts
¼ cup raw almonds
¾ cup raw cacao powder
½ cup unsweetened shredded coconut
pinch of sea salt
2 tablespoons cold water
1 tablespoon vanilla extract

Line a 20cm x 20cm square cake tin with baking paper.

Place the dates, nuts, cacao powder, coconut and salt in a food processor, and process until the dates and nuts are coarsely chopped.

Add the water and vanilla extract, and process until the mixture is moist but not sticky.

Press very firmly into the prepared tin, then cover with cling film and refrigerate for at least one hour before cutting into bars. Keep bars refrigerated for up to one week.

SECTION 2
LIVE LEAN

13. EXERCISE
THE OTHER HALF
OF THE EQUATION

OK, cool — if you have read the first bit of this book you will now know the basic nutritional framework you need to follow in order to provide your body with the optimal nutrition or fuel. In this section you will learn how to put that fuel to use and improve your health further through physical conditioning and exercise. This is the stuff that will make you unstoppable!

Your body needs to move. It's designed to move. Human beings are animals, and just like our animal cousins, our bodies want to be active. We are built to bend and stretch, to run and jump and lift and pull. Our muscles and joints, circulatory system, internal organs and, perhaps most importantly, our brains, all need the benefits of regular exercise to keep them in tip-top form.

So throw this book on the ground and run outside! No, actually, just keep reading and learn a bit more about it and *then* do that.

Exercise is a very broad term and incorporates any form of physical activity. Walking, running, dancing, lifting weights, playing sport, jumping on your bed — whatever it is, if it involves sustained physical exertion and movement, then it's exercise.

Fitness is also a very broad term, but basically I like to think of it as your physical health or condition resulting from any sort of exercise and movement. Cardiovascular fitness, muscular strength, muscular endurance and flexibility are all types of fitness. The tool that we use to improve and influence our fitness is exercise.

MY EXERCISE JOURNEY

Earlier I told you a bit about how I came to adopt a paleo lifestyle, and the various 'experiments' I conducted to work out what the best eating regime was for my body. While not to the same extent, I did a similar thing with exercise, and have tried a variety of different plans and types of exercise before finding what I think is the best regime for all-round fitness and good health (if you just want to get to the nitty-gritty, skip to page 264).

I've always been very active. As I've said, I grew up on a farm and used to come home from school and just run around. We didn't have a TV until I was about seven so my sister and I used to make our own fun outside.

My dad was a very physical guy, into his exercise as well as working on the farm, and I grew up really looking up to him in terms of how he kept himself fit and healthy. He played rugby when I was young and I remember hanging out down at the rugby club at weekends with the other kids, eating lollies, chips and Fanta, and running off the sugar high. As I mentioned earlier, Dad had a home-made gym in the garage and I used to watch him lifting his tractor-axle-and-drench-container weights and try to copy him.

When I was at primary school I played a lot of sport, and got into tennis, rugby, soccer and badminton. At high school I added touch rugby and started getting into athletics in quite a big way. I started exercising in a structured, purposeful way and catered the training I did around competing in track and field, specifically high jump, triple jump, 400 metres and javelin. I was competing in inter-school and club competitions and I found having a goal like building up for a major competition kept me focused.

A lot of people drop their sport when they leave school to go on to tertiary education or full-time work, since the opportunities aren't so easily presented to you and life gets in the way. But it was always really important to me, and when I moved to Dunedin to go to uni I carried on with my athletics, soccer and rugby. I played for a law-school rugby team, and a semi-competitive soccer team called the Purple Cobras with a bunch of mates — it was a good blend of competition and fun. I also started taking my athletics more seriously, especially javelin. I began training for javelin a few times a week with my coach, Raylene Bates, and for the first time started to train my body specifically for one event. I learnt so much about sport-specific training from Raylene, and found that focusing on this discipline really helped my overall fitness — it made me strong, powerful and fast, and improved my performance in my other sports (namely rugby). I was going to the gym and doing a couple of sessions a week, concentrating on my legs and core strength, plus some technique and throwing sessions.

At the time I was also studying sports science, so it was interesting to be able to apply what I was learning in a practical environment. It also helped me to understand how the exercise I was doing was affecting my body, and the mechanisms behind health and fitness. This helped me to figure out why I should do certain exercises, and the best way of doing them to produce maximum results. For example, if someone just told you to do 50 squats, you might not be motivated to do them because you wouldn't really know why you'd be doing them, other than for the reason that everyone says squats are important. But, if that person sat down with you and explained to you what's happening in your body when you do these squats and what benefits you're going to get out of doing them, you'd probably be a bit more motivated and interested in doing them.

In the end my best result in javelin was a third at the national athletics championships. I would have liked to have gone on doing it, but I knew I was never going to be New Zealand's best javelin thrower, or go to the Olympics or Commonwealth Games. Plus I moved up to Auckland once I finished my degree, away from my coach, and into the real world — as I'm sure many graduates can relate to — so it was time to move on.

I spent a couple of seasons coaching tennis in the United States before going to Western Australia to work managing a gym at a mining camp (for more on this, see page 11). It was the first time I had really used my degree practically in employment, applying what I had learnt at uni in a physical fitness environment.

As I mentioned earlier, it also gave me lots of time, while the miners were off mining, to work on my own fitness. I had a great opportunity to work out as much as I wanted and get super fit. It was a pretty sweet gig, getting to work out all the time, but I guess there really wasn't much else to do in the outback. At times I would get pretty bored so I would give myself little workout challenges or do exercise experiments. One time in the middle of summer. I decided to see how much I could sweat in one hour, so I weighed myself before and after an hour of running and hill sprints in the scorching sun (usually temperatures were in the 40s!). It's quite easy to figure out because 1 litre of water (or sweat) weighs 1 kilogram. At the post-run weigh-in I had lost almost 3 kilograms — that's 3 litres of sweat! And then about half an hour later I got a migraine. I decided not to do that experiment again.

As I was doing with my diet, I tried out all sorts of different workout regimes and did lots of reading and research about exercise techniques. There are so many different types of exercise and schools of thought about what is best that you could try a different routine or type of exercise every day for a year and still have stuff left to try! Plus there are different training techiques to achieve different results, such as doing fewer reps (repetitions) with heavy weights if you want to build muscle and more reps with lighter weights if you want to tone without getting bigger.

The key thing, I found, was not necessarily *what* I was doing but *how* I was doing it. Whatever fitness regime you follow, every time you work out you need to go as hard as you can. I realised that if I really wanted to see results and changes I needed to push myself to the absolute max every time — no coasting or going easy on myself. I even had a motto in my gym which I wrote on all the clocks: 'No time for weakness'. A little corny but it helped me push myself.

So many people at the gym at the mine would ask me to write them a programme, and then I would see them come in and just go leisurely through the motions. Then they'd come back and say, 'I'm not getting the results I thought I would.' This was due to a combination of things: firstly, these people were impatient and expected results immediately (hence why many shortcuts were taken, including taking steriods and fat-burning drugs); and secondly, sure they were doing the exercises and the right number of reps, but they weren't pushing themselves. They would just meander through the workout, never upping the intensity (by increasing the weight or reps) or their effort, and they'd leave the gym without having even worked up a sweat! Probably the biggest thing I learnt from my time at the gym in Australia was that if you want results you've got to put in the effort, be patient and know that results will come.

I also found what I consider to be the ideal type of exercise for the human body — something called functional body-weight fitness training, which uses simple, everyday movements and body weight alone to build strength, muscle and improve cardiovascular fitness. It is now the core of my exercise regime, and it's the basis for the exercises I share with you in chapter 21.

But first, let's take a look at why exercise is so important.

MY FITNESS WEEK

Now I am back in New Zealand and working full time, I don't have the luxury of working out whenever I feel like it. However, I still try to incorporate a range of different exercise opportunities into my week, making sure I always get some exercise every day.

Most weekday mornings I am up at 5.30am to do a workout at Ludus Magnus before work. Ludus Magnus is what got me interested in functional fitness. It's a gym and community where you do fitness classes predominantly involving body-weight exercises, and you just go as hard as you like (see page 263). At the time of writing this though, I am also doing a few boxing training sessions a week, building up for a charity boxing event. If I can find time, I do try to fit in a traditional weights workout at the gym once a week as well, concentrating on my legs and a little bit of upper-body work.

But, for my general fitness, ease of movement, everyday functionality, flexibility and strength, I believe functional fitness exercises are the best.

I also play indoor netball for a social team in the winter, and touch rugby in the summer, along with a bit of tennis. I find social sports to be so good for me mentally — they're fun and social, and I'm exercising without really knowing it.

At the weekends I try to incorporate exercise into my leisure time, maybe going for a walk, a run or a bike ride with friends.

14. WHY EXERCISE?

Being active is one of the most important things you can do for your health. I believe everyone should do some form of exercise every single day, even if it's just walking at least part of the way to work from your car or the bus, or walking round the block at lunchtime. Too many people's lives these days follow the same routine: get up, sit in the car, sit down at work in front of the computer, sit in the car and drive home, sit down and watch TV, go to bed and sleep, then wake up and do it all again, all while eating too much of the wrong food. Basically, that's just shortening your potential lifespan and making you unhappy and overweight! Regular exercise will not only make your body feel better, it will improve your mental wellbeing and overall quality of life.

If you are truly committed to being as healthy as possible, through eating as healthily as possible, then you need to back it up with exercise. There is no point in thinking about what you're eating while you're sitting on your arse.

I find that eating well makes me want to exercise, and vice versa. The last thing I feel like after a workout is some unhealthy pile of junk food. And then when I eat healthily I find that I have more energy for exercise. It's like my body is telling me to continue improving its health.

As well as releasing endorphins that give you a feeling of pleasure and contentment after you exercise, there are also longer-term mental-health benefits. Put pretty simply, exercise makes you feel good about yourself. It gives you a sense of achievement and makes you feel more positive. And, if you are exercising regularly, you are going to look good, and this is going to give you confidence and make you feel unstoppable. It's a virtuous cycle: you do something good for yourself and it makes you feel good, so you do more of it. You look good, so you keep up the good work. *Boom!* Welcome to the health cycle.

Here is some more good news about exercise.

→ Everyone knows this one, but it's worth repeating: exercise is great for your cardiovascular system (your heart and lungs, and their ability to get oxygenated blood around your body). Cardiovascular disease (heart, stroke and blood-vessel disease) is still the leading cause of death in New Zealand, accounting for a shocking 30 per cent of deaths annually. The Heart Foundation estimates that, on average, a New Zealander dies from heart disease *every 90 minutes*. WTF! That's insane, right? And it's not just men dying: in 2012, an average of 60 Kiwi women died of heart disease every week.

→ Exercise helps reduce cholesterol levels (improve your blood lipid profile), and helps regulate your blood pressure and blood-sugar levels — all important factors in avoiding chronic disease.

→ Reducing your body fat, especially the level of visceral fat in your abdomen around your organs, reduces your risk of chronic diseases, such as diabetes, some cancers and even dementia.

→ Increased muscle mass increases your overall metabolism, so the fitter and stronger you are, the more efficient your body is at burning food for energy rather than storing it as fat.

→ Being functionally fit and having strong muscles and active joints means you are less susceptible to injury. You can take part in everyday activities easily and comfortably, without wondering if your body is going to hold up! Bending, lifting, climbing, carrying, walking up stairs with a spring in your step . . . Having good core strength also means you are less likely to hurt your back, which is the second most common reason for people taking time off work for sickness or injury.

→ Exercise is also good for your brain. As well as the short-term effects of the release of endorphins (feel-good chemicals) during and after exercise, studies have shown that regular exercise improves cognitive function and may help to ward off or slow the effects of dementia in later life. Now that's something to remember . . . or not.

→ As well as that short-term rush, exercise has been shown to have positive effects on longer-term mental health, reducing depression and anxiety. The National Depression Initiative (see depression. org.nz) says doing regular physical activity is likely to be helpful even for quite severe depression. I know that whenever I'm feeling down or stressed for whatever reason if I do some exercise it really turns me around.

→ Exercise has a positive effect on your immunity. Researchers aren't quite sure why, but regular moderate exercise seems to improve the human immune system and make us less susceptible to viruses and bacteria.

→ Scientific studies also suggest that regular exercise will help you to sleep better (see page 334 for why that's so important). Multiple studies have shown that exercise improves overall sleep time and increases slow-wave sleep time (considered important for body repair and maintenance).

→ And here's the real clincher: exercise is good for your sex life. Multiple studies show that regular exercise improves sexual function and enjoyment by improving the cardiovascular system and improving circulation to all the important bits. For guys, it can lower your risk of erectile dysfunction, reduce your chances of getting a condition called

BPH, which causes the prostate gland to become enlarged, and improve your sperm count. (A study in the *British Journal of Sports Medicine* showed that men who watched more than 20 hours of TV per week had considerably lower sperm counts than those who watched no TV.) Bar yourself up with exercise. And for girls there are benefits too — improving circulation, releasing endorphins and lowering stress levels.

Plus, it's now cool to be healthy. No one looks at someone out for a run or heading to the gym and thinks, 'What a loser.' No one's going to give you a hard time for looking after yourself. Sure, some people might get into oversharing their workouts on social media, but by and large it's a great thing to see people being proud of being fit and healthy.

LENGTHEN YOUR LIFE
ԼԼԼԼ

Now, I have no idea how they figure this out, but the New Zealand Heart Foundation says that, for every hour of exercise you do, you gain about two hours of additional life expectancy. I like this stat. Let's apply it: say you did on average an hour of exercise five days a week for a year (which is doable) then you would add an extra 21.5 days to your life. Cool — extra life! I'll have that thanks.

15. WHAT EXERCISE IS RIGHT FOR ME?

....

Every single person can benefit from exercise. What type of exercise you decide to do depends on your goals and values. Someone who wants to lose weight is going to benefit more from a different type of exercise to someone who wants to gain muscle. If you want to increase flexibility, you'd choose something like yoga and stretches.

If I had to say what type of exercise is most beneficial to the majority of people, I would say functional body-weight fitness. You can tailor it to your own goals and the intensity at which you want to exercise. You don't need special equipment, you don't need a gym membership, you can do it anywhere and any time. (See more on functional fitness in chapter 18.)

RESISTANCE

The critical factor in all forms of exercise is resistance. The reason your body needs some form of resistance when exercising — that is, your muscles have to produce some effort — is so that it knows it needs to adapt to meet the challenge. If you are lifting heavy weights (providing high resistance) your body will get the message that it needs to make your muscles bigger and stronger so you can do more of this type of work. If you are lifting lighter weights, or doing light body-weight exercises, it knows to make the existing muscles stronger and more toned, but not neccesarily bigger, so they can perform efficiently. When you do cardio, your body improves the efficiency of your heart and lungs to make sure plenty of oxygenated blood can get to where it's needed.

If your goal is to lose weight then, as well as paying careful attention to your nutrition, I would recommend running, swimming, biking or rowing on a machine. But I would do this as a supplement to a core programme of functional body-weight fitness exercises. Swimming is a great addition to your fitness regime, and is much easier on your joints than running. It is especially good if you are recovering from an injury. Stationary rowing is an excellent cardio and strength exercise, but is not for you if you have any back issues as the body position required for rowing does put stress on your lower back.

If your goal is cardiovascular fitness and endurance — maybe you want to do a running event, or you need to be cardio fit for your job or hobby, such as sailing — you might want to add running to your workout schedule. I didn't used to like running but now I love it. It's a great cardiovascular workout that gets your heart and lungs going for a solid period of time, plus I find it really good mentally — it helps to clear my head, gives me some thinking space and of course, like all exercise, releases endorphins that impart a sense of wellbeing. You never feel worse after going for a run (unless you roll your ankle or slip over in dog shit). It's especially good if you add some interval training — instead of running at a steady pace the whole time, challenge yourself to some blocks of short sprints within the run.

Unless you have a particular goal of doing a marathon or half-marathon, then you don't have to be running long distances to get the benefits. The physical impact of long-distance running can be hard on your joints, and I know that in the past when I have trained for a half-marathon I have developed sore knees. The longest run I would do now would be no more than 10 kilometres. Generally a good distance to run is between 5 and 7 kilometres, or for about 30 or 40 minutes.

Cycling is another popular choice, and with very good reason — it's low impact, great cardio and tones your legs. It's probably more practical in some places than others: the big thing that puts me off cycling in Auckland is the traffic and the dismal safety record of cyclists on our roads! Another option if you are into cycling is spin classes (indoor cycling), which keeps you off the roads and motivated by a group-exercise environment, an instructor and good music. I used to do spin classes a lot, and found they made me sweat more than any other form of exercise.

Group fitness classes are worth a go if they are not already 'your thing'. Check out what your local gym or leisure centre is offering in terms of step classes, dance- or sports-based classes, regimes using hand weights and classes that incorporate yoga or Pilates moves. I enjoy doing classes because of the social aspect — it's fun to work out in a group and it helps to keep me motivated. It makes me feel like part of a team. I like the community aspect of going to the gym and getting to know other people, and finding out about their fitness journey and goals. They might have different aims, strengths and interests, but we're all challenging ourselves and taking on the workout. And I know it's a bit clichéd, but it's 100 per cent true: the limiting factor is not our bodies, it's our minds, and what we think we can and cannot do.

If dancing is your thing, you might be motivated by Zumba or a hip-hop based class. And don't worry about not being able to keep up or learn the moves — it's just fun to try, and you'll soon get the hang of it. Also, remember that no one else is watching you — they're too busy trying to bust their own moves or watching themselves in the mirror! Fitness classes can be really motivating — it's much harder to stop and take a breather when everyone else is moving around you,

NO LIGHTS NO LYCRA

ееее

If you want to dance like no one's watching, find out if there's a No Lights No Lycra group near you — there are groups in the four main centres and some provincial areas too (see nolightsnolycra.com). No Lights No Lycra was set up by a group of Australian dance students in 2009 and offers a space for people to dance however they like in the dark, usually in a community-hall-type place. There are no instructors, no set moves and no judgement, just good music and a social atmosphere. I've been a couple of times and have friends that go regularly — it's great fun and a good way to exercise, like dancing around your living room but with a whole lot of other like-minded people. Look it up if you think it might be your gig.

and there's a real atmosphere generated by a roomful of people producing endorphins and having fun.

If you want to add strength and flexibility to your exercise regime, definitely explore yoga and Pilates. As well as toning your body, opening and loosening your joints, and improving your flexibility, yoga is fantastic for your mental state. Breathing is a critical part of yoga practice, and learning this skill can help massively with stress relief and relaxation. Pilates is also fantastic for core strength and flexibility, and can hugely improve your posture and physical functionality. I injured my back quite badly a few years ago, so bought a book on Pilates and began implementing the movements and workouts to strengthen my core and back. I put my rapid recovery down to using these techniques.

WHAT ABOUT WORKING WITH A PERSONAL TRAINER?

Is it worth spending a whole lot of money to get someone to personally kick your butt several times a week? I would have to say, for the average person, the answer is no. But, in saying that, I know that having a PT does work well for some people, and a couple of my friends say that without a PT they wouldn't exercise at all. Having a PT makes them accountable to someone, and having to pay their PT means they take their exercise more seriously. However, unless you have a disposable income that allows for this investment — or you're a celebrity, in which case it appears to be a necessity — having a PT is an unsustainable luxury.

A lot of people sign up with a PT because they think it'll be an easy option: they can just do what they're told and sit back and relax the rest of the time. A good PT will really push their client, and might even make you work harder than you would make yourself! But, unless you really need someone to push you or the idea of an unbreakable appointment and getting your money's worth to get you motivated, I don't think you need a PT.

It's good to have someone who can give you ideas

and exercises, but if you belong to a gym the instructors there should be able to help you. That was the kind of work I did in Australia — setting gym programmes, giving advice and answering questions — and it should be part of your gym membership. Or just jump on the computer and do a bit of research — chances are most trainers will have gained a lot of their exercise regimes, techniques and ideas from the internet anyway.

If what you need is a way to make a commitment to exercise, you can get the same effect by doing a regular class or working out with a friend, at a fraction of the cost. Having a workout buddy is probably the number-one thing that helps people stick to exercising regularly.

➤ TIP: Making a commitment to exercise is a matter of prioritising your health. So often we prioritise work, or friends and family, or other commitments, above looking after ourselves. Keeping yourself fit and healthy should be one of your biggest priorities. You're no use to friends and family if you're sick, and no one on their death bed ever says, 'I wish I'd spent more time at work.' Think about your priorities and the quality of life that you desire, and make regular exercise a non-negotiable in your life.

And, before you tell me you don't have time to exercise, remember this: Barack Obama finds time to work out every day, and he's probably got a lot more on than you or me.

SOCIAL SPORTS

Playing social sports with a team of friends or workmates is a great way to exercise and have fun at the same time. Indoor netball, cricket and soccer are all great workouts and give you an excuse to hang out with your mates afterwards. Just watch the after-match beers.

EXERCISE AND WEIGHT LOSS

If you are wanting to lose weight, then 80 per cent of this will be down to what you eat, not the exercise you do. It is much easier to adjust the amount of energy going into the body than increase energy out to make up for everything you are eating. However, exercise is the other 20 per cent and will provide you with all the benefits mentioned on the previous pages as well as contributing to your weight loss.

If you want to lose weight, functional body-weight fitness can be the best way to do it. If you enjoy running and cardio then also include as much of that as you want, or even just walking. However, from a calorie-burning point of view, you will burn far more calories doing a high-intensity strength workout which doubles as a cardio workout if you don't rest as much. People don't traditionally think of resistance exercises as a way to lose weight because of the way they are traditionally done: do ten repetitions, then rest, then do another ten. But, if you do ten squats then ten push-ups then

MAKING IT FUN

~~~~

I still play tennis, touch and indoor netball, like I did when I was a teenager. When you're younger, you exercise a lot without even thinking about it: running around the playground, climbing and chasing your mates (or the girls). There are so many opportunities to be physically active at school, during and after class, that you don't even realise you're exercising.

To maximise your enjoyment of exercise as an adult, choose something you find fun. If you like riding a bike, go for bike rides with friends or do spin classes. Don't like running? Don't run (although I'd say give it a try if you used to hate it when you were younger — it can be great stress relief, and you might surprise yourself and enjoy it). Play a team sport with your mates, or a racquet sport against them. Go to a fitness class and feel the energy surge you get from exercising in a group. Team up with someone at the gym to keep you motivated.

I think it's great to combine exercise and socialising, whether you're playing a team sport or training with a buddy. Exercising with someone else will increase your enjoyment and your motivation. Plus, on those days when you feel like you can't be bothered working out, if you have an 'appointment' with a buddy, you'll be less likely to pike out.

ten chin-ups, then do that three times, and rest as little as possible, you'll be breathing hard and doing a cardio workout too. Time yourself and then, to challenge yourself, see if you can do the next ten of each exercise more quickly. Think about keeping your heart rate elevated.

WOMEN AND WEIGHTS

Some women are reluctant to do weights and other resistance exercise because they don't want to get big and muscly. However, it is physiologically much more difficult for women to build muscle than it is for men, due to hormonal differences, so you seriously needn't worry about this. Women have lower levels of testosterone and higher levels of body fat, which means with resistance exercise their muscles become stronger and more toned without becoming bulky.

You are likely to get some serious muscle if you're doing full-on weightlifting or CrossFit, however, as that has quite a large weightlifting component (see opposite page). But for women to achieve these big muscles it takes an incredible amount of effort, motivation and resistance. CrossFit has helped to popularise the muscly, strong look for women, and these women are justifiably proud of their bodies. If that's your goal, go for it.

WHAT ABOUT CROSSFIT?

Paleo and CrossFit often seem to go together, especially in the United States, where the CrossFit workout system was developed. The official 'dietary prescription' for CrossFit is similar to the paleo lifestyle: lean protein, low-GI carbohydrates, healthy fat, little starch and no sugar.

So, what is CrossFit? Well, it's an exercise regime that is also based on Olympic weightlifting and the functional fitness philosophy — that is, based on the body's core natural movements — but includes additional weights over and above body weight. It's kind of like competitive weight training, combining aspects of weightlifting, high-intensity interval training, plyometrics (using explosive jump-type movements to increase strength), gymnastics and calisthenics (body-weight exercises) to give you both a strength and a cardio workout at the same time. It's held in a class format, including a challenging WOD, or Workout of the Day, so you are motivated by both the instructor and your peers. It's not just a workout, either; there are CrossFit competitions, too, where enthusiasts compete against each other to complete workout combinations. The basic theory, according to CrossFit.com, is: 'A regimen of constantly varied, functional movements performed at high intensity in a communal environment [that] leads to health and fitness.'

CrossFit was developed in the US by trainer Greg Glassman, and started to become popular in the early

2000s. Now they reckon there is a worldwide network of around 11,000 affiliated gyms and more than 100,000 trainers. It has been in New Zealand since 2008, and has grown massively in popularity over the past few years.

A lot of people love it, and it meets their needs perfectly: keeping them motivated and giving them both a strength and cardio workout. The community aspect is really important too — it's easy to get caught up in the hype of WODs, personal bests and sharing your successes with others in the group, and gyms often organise social events too. It's aimed at people who want to get strong, fit and muscly, and it creates a certain type of body. (I can spot a CrossFitter pretty easily.) If you want to be big, doing CrossFit regularly will probably work for you.

But is it just the next exercise fad, which will come and go? I don't think so, but I do think it will start to plateau. It's not for everyone — it's intense, it isn't cheap and it doesn't suit everyone's fitness goals.

I personally don't think it's that good for your body, and it doesn't meet my goals of being strong and lean without being overly big. The movements, especially the weightlifting stuff, put a lot of stress on your joints, and I think that the weights can be too heavy for some people. The competitiveness aspect can be quite positive and motivating, and some people really respond to that and push themselves hard. But for some people, including myself, this means a lower focus on form and safety.

I injured my back doing CrossFit, getting all

competitive on the WOD. Everyone watches how well you do, and I like to do well. Anyway, the WOD involved a clean-and-press aspect (an Olympic lift involving lifting a weighted bar from the ground up and over your head). About halfway through the WOD I was more focused on smashing out the reps of the clean and press than I was on form and safety. Because I was warmed up I just felt a little twinge in my back and didn't think anything of it. Big mistake. It wasn't until the next morning that I realised I could hardly move. In fact, I had a prolapsed spinal disc and spent months having physio to get it right again. Even after a few years it is still prone to re-injury.

Obviously, this doesn't happen to everyone, but I do feel that the potential is there. I just don't think it's necessary to put your body under such extreme stress and strain so as to be optimally healthy or to reach fitness goals. You can get just as good a result doing functional body-weight fitness exercises without additional weights, and without the intensely competitive aspect.

I also think CrossFit develops quite a narrow range of fitness. For example, a CrossFitter typically isn't going to be a great runner because their muscle mass is too great for them to be able to run efficiently and economically. I want to be the fastest, strongest and most efficiently adapted to as many types of exercise as I can be. I want to be flexible and have good joint mobility. I want to be strong and explosive so that I can be fast and powerful. I want to be fit and economical so that I can run with ease. I want to be able to run

and jump around on the netball court without getting injured. And I want to live in a healthy body that will keep me going for many years to come. These are the reasons why I largely prefer to work out using my body weight only.

16. WHAT'S YOUR MOTIVATION?

I'm lucky. I don't usually have any trouble getting motivated to exercise. But, like everyone, I do have my bad days, when I need to remind myself to get out there and get moving. So, if you need some good reasons to exercise, here's what keeps me going.

→ I enjoy feeling fit and healthy. I like the feeling that I am treating my body well and giving it what it needs, and in exchange it is working at its optimum. I feel as if I'm always working to create a perfect machine.

→ I like the endorphin rush and stress relief I get from working out, going for a run or playing sport. It's a great way to shake off stress or the busyness of the day.

→ I like the social aspect of playing sport or doing

a fitness class, spending time doing something positive with like-minded people.

→ I am competitive, and I like satisfying that urge by playing well or doing a good workout. Even if I'm just competing against myself to better a workout time, do a few more reps or exercise for longer, I still like to win!

→ I like to look good. Let's be honest, we all like to look lean and healthy. And it doesn't happen without putting in a bit of effort. Being happy with how I look helps me feel confident and gives me a good outlook on life.

→ I sometimes give myself fitness goals. Previously I have entered events, such as Tough Mudder, a half-marathon, and the Sky Tower Stair Challenge, for which I have needed to train to reach my goal of nailing them. At the moment I'm doing boxing training — my motivation is that if I don't train enough there is a chance I will get punched in the face heaps of times, and I don't really like the idea of that!

Figure out what makes you feel motivated to exercise and take advantage of it. Set some goals (see chapter 17) and get ready to enjoy the results.

THE PRESSURE TO LOOK GOOD

Whether you admit it or not, everyone wants to look good. We all look at other people and compare ourselves to them from time to time, and sometimes think, 'Wow, I'd like to look like that.' The media and society put a lot of pressure on both guys and girls to look good — although the definition of 'good' is very changeable, subjective and sometimes not very attainable or even desirable from a health point of view. I know it can be a huge pressure for women, but it's become an increasing source of anxiety for men as well. For women the ideal generally seems to be being slim, and it has been for decades. There has also been a movement in recent years towards a big booty being a desirable physical attribute — mental images of Kim Kardashian and Nicki Minaj bounce into my mind. For guys it's being big — strong and muscly with not much body fat, similar to a fitness model.

Trying to get a body like that isn't realistic for many people. Their genetics simply wont allow it, no matter how many squats or sit-ups they do. Futhermore, in some cases, those models or celebrities may not actually be very healthy at all from an overall body-health point of view. But, if striving to look like an 'ideal' makes you feel good about yourself, then go for it! Just make sure you're doing it safely and healthily, and don't get disheartened if you don't achieve the ideal — many are not at all realistic.

My personal ideal, and the state I try to strive for, is looking muscular, lean — so, not carrying unnecessary body fat — and healthy. I believe the paleo lifestyle helps me to achieve this, by keeping my body lean and making me look healthy overall through having plenty of exercise, good food and sleep (see chapter 22 for more on the importance of sleep).

The most important thing is being happy with how you look and feel. If you know you are treating your body right, with the right food and exercise, then your actual shape doesn't matter. You will have a healthy, functional body that you can be proud of.

And remember, if you're not happy with how your body looks, change it. The body can adapt; it just takes some time and a bunch of effort.

17. GOALS
SETTING THEM AND STICKING TO THEM

..............•

Exercise is usually performed because of a goal, and that goal determines the type of exercise. For example, if your goal is to improve your cardiovascular fitness or compete in a fun run or distance event, you go for a run; if your goal is to have big muscles to impress the girls at the beach this summer, you lift big weights; or if your goal is to improve your flexibility you might do a bunch of stretches or take up yoga. Generally all types of exercise will help you lose weight when you are eating the right food — again, if that is one of your goals.

From time to time I make specific fitness goals by training for an event or competition of some sort, but for many years now I have really just had one overarching goal: to be the fittest and healthiest I can be, through diet and exercise. This goal is always at the back of my mind and it influences my life every day — it's in my mind every time I decide what to eat or what I'm going to do in terms of exercise.

If you are starting out on your health and fitness journey, it will really help if you have specific, clear, measurable goals. It might be to lose a certain amount of weight or body fat, or to run or cycle a certain distance, or to improve your strength, your cardio fitness or your flexibility. The key for any type of goal is to make it challenging, so that you will experience a positive change, but it also needs to be achievable.

If you don't set yourself clear, achievable goals, it's much harder to tell if you are making progress and therefore motivate yourself to keep going. Working towards a competitive event like a 5-kilometre or 10-kilometre run or a half-marathon can be a good goal, but you need to continue to motivate yourself up to that event. A good way to do that is to set smaller 'milestone' goals that you achieve along the way and will help you to reach your end goal.

Let's take that half-marathon as an example. Your end goal is to run a half-marathon — 21.1 kilometres — as fast as you can. For this you might set some milestone goals like running non-stop for 40 minutes, then an hour, then an hour and a half; or running non-stop for 10 kilometres, then 14 kilometres, then 17 kilometres. Whatever these milestone goals are, they will help you in your journey and keep you motivated to reach that end goal of running a half-marathon in a good time.

And then, once you complete this end goal, you may even realise that this is itself a milestone goal — a step along the way to creating your healthiest body and life possible.

Once you are happy with your state of health, in terms of diet and exercise, you will find your body will give you clear feedback if it's not getting what it needs or wants. I track my ongoing goal to be as healthy and fit as possible by how my body reacts. If I don't eat the right things, exercise enough, have too much stress or don't get adequate sleep, I feel shit, simple as that. I know that, generally, if I am feeling good, full of energy and positive I am doing the right things.

SOME TIPS FOR SETTING GOALS

→ Make them realistic. If you decide you want to lose 20 kilograms over the course of a year, that's doable. If you want to lose it for your friend's wedding in four weeks' time — not going to happen. Don't set yourself up for failure, because no one likes to fail. Plus, if you are continually failing to meet your unrealistic goals, you're more likely to just give up on trying to make improvements to your life. Success breeds success, so make sure you set realistic goals and celebrate achieving them.

→ Write them down. Stick them on the fridge or somewhere you will see them and be reminded of them regularly. It's always good to have your goals in mind.

→ Share your goals with friends and family — it gives you someone else to be accountable to. Let them know what you hope to achieve and discuss your progress with them. It will help you to stay motivated and true to your word.

→ Check in with your goals regularly and track your progress. Set up a chart or a spreadsheet (if you're into that sort of thing) and record how you're going. This is also great for seeing how far you've come and reflecting on the progress you've made.

→ Break big goals down into smaller milestone goals, so you feel like you are making progress. Track your weight loss over time. Aim to be eating paleo 50 per cent of the time, then 60, then 70. Go for one week without processed sugar, then two or three. It's like eating an elephant: if you had to eat the whole thing at once, it'd be impossible, but if you ate it piece by piece, day by day, you'd get there in the end. (OK, that's a pretty weird analogy, but it does kind of make sense.)

→ Reward yourself. No, not with a big piece of chocolate cake. But celebrate your successes in other ways — time with friends, a movie, something you really enjoy. (The odd drink now and then isn't too bad to reward yourself with — just make sure you're not rewarding yourself this way every day.)

→ Have a strong motivation for your goal. Learn more about the benefits of healthy diet and exercise, so that on days when you really can't be bothered being 'good' you can remind yourself of all the benefits:

longer life, better sleep, more admiring looks as you walk along the beach, being better in bed, being better than your friends at sport, whatever.

→ Give yourself a break. No one moves towards success in an even, straight line — it's more like an up-and-down zig-zag. But as long as the overall progress is in the right direction, don't beat yourself up if you waver a little.

GOAL WEIGHT
ℓℓℓℓ

One of the most common health and fitness goals is setting a goal weight that you want to achieve. While this is a worthy goal, it might not be that simple. As discussed on page 126, deciding on what is a healthy weight for your body and build can be difficult. The BMI will give you an idea, but is not a reliable measure.

I think a better indicator is body-fat percentage. Being lean and not carrying unnecessary body fat is important to me, and I know it has a more significant impact on my health than keeping my overall weight down.

I also think it's more about what you look like, how your clothes fit and how you feel than trying to aim for some specific goal weight. By all means set a goal, or perhaps an upper and lower limit within which you want to sit, but don't be a slave to the scales. It all comes down to feeling good about yourself when you look in the mirror.

18. FUNCTIONAL BODY-WEIGHT FITNESS

·············•

As part of my fitness journey, I tried all sorts of different forms of exercise, workout regimes and sports. But the one I think works best for me is functional body-weight fitness. Body-weight exercises are great for gaining strength, building muscle, boosting cardiovascular fitness, losing weight and improving flexibility. These exercises don't cost you anything and can be performed anywhere — all you need is your body.

I like this style of exercise because there is something natural about using just your body to work on your body. The modern-day paleo lifestyle aims to replicate a period when people were naturally active all the time, and this style of exercise is highly appropriate from that perspective, as it mimics natural physical movements.

Functional fitness is practical and appropriate for the needs of everyday life. It's doing the things your body is designed to do — bending, lifting, carrying, jumping. It's safer than doing weights as you never have to lift anything other than your own body weight, plus you don't have to go to the gym to do it. You can do it at home, at work, when you're travelling — anywhere there's enough space to swing a cat (if you hate cats). You don't need any special equipment besides a bar for doing body-weight pulling exercises (like pull-ups), and you can make the workout as long or short or hard or easy as you want (just don't make it too easy, or you won't achieve anything).

The exercises can be modified to any fitness level and any age. Whether you're a beginner or an elite athlete, you will reap the benefits. Adding repetitions, or performing the exercises faster or super slowly are a few ways to make even the simplest exercises more challenging.

Since body-weight exercises use no weights, increasing resistance is accomplished in other ways. For example, a push-up can be ramped up by swapping it for a clap push-up, or a lunge can be made harder by doing a jumping lunge. Depending on what your fitness goals are, you can easily adjust your body-weight workouts accordingly. And progress is easy to measure since body-weight exercises offer tons of ways to do a little more in each workout.

Because cardiovascular fitness is also important for overall good health, you can either combine functional body-weight fitness with a cardio workout like running or cycling, or you can add a cardio aspect to your workout by doing increased repetitions at higher speed, and by resting less in between sets. This way you keep your heart rate up, so you are essentially doing cardio and resistance training at the same time. Saves a bit of time, eh?

As I said above, I see so many people at the gym doing a set of reps on a machine then spending ages walking around, chatting to a mate, having a drink and letting themselves cool down before starting the next set. That's OK if you're lifting very heavy weights and trying to gain large muscle, but it's kind of wasting your time and effort if you are trying to improve your overall fitness.

Functional body-weight fitness exercise is part of a wider movement towards simplifying exercise and getting back to basics, using body weight. A lot of gyms are now running classes that focus on body-weight exercises.

GLADIATOR TRAINING

One of the places I like to work out is an Auckland gym called Ludus Magnus. It's a functional fitness gym which takes its name from the Great Gladiatorial Training School in Rome. That may sound a bit intense, but it's not really — it just involves a lot of fast-paced body-weight fitness and functional movements. We do use a few small weights called kettlebells, which are like a cannonball with a handle on the top, but generally it is about using the weight of your own body to provide resistance. That means lots of squats, lunges, push-ups, chin-ups, animal crawls and burpees. (For more on these types of exercises, see chapter 19.)

19. THE EXERCISES

.... •

In the following section I outline what I believe is the best type of exercise for improving fitness in every aspect, at every level. I have given you the framework to be able to structure your own exercise to suit your own body (because every body is different) and to reach your own goals — whether your goal is to lose weight, build and/or tone muscle, or just to create the fittest and healthiest body possible.

Over the next pages I will give you 30 basic exercises, covering your legs, chest and shoulders, abdominals and back, arms and full body. Then I have included a series of 24 workouts, which are combinations of the basic exercises to work your whole body. You can also mix and match your own combinations to suit your goals, or areas you want to work out and focus on.

As a general rule, the more reps of an exercise you do, the better it will be for improving cardio and muscular endurance and toning. Doing fewer reps that require more effort because they have greater resistance (are harder to perform) will result in improvements to muscular strength and muscle hypertrophy (an increase in the size of the muscle). No matter what, though, if you are trying hard, sweating and getting your heart rate up, any variations, level and form of these exercises is going to help you lose body fat.

With body-weight exercises it is important to continue to push and challenge yourself physically and mentally as you get fitter. After a while of performing some of the exercises at a certain level of difficulty or intensity you may find your progress starts to slow down. To keep making improvements you must challenge yourself to perform more difficult variations to improve your performance. For example, if you can perform flawless sets of squats, you must challenge yourself to perform a more difficult variation, such as jump squats (see page 270) or pistol squats (see page 277). If you're finding a regular burpee a bit easy after a while, have a go at a clap burpee.

HOW TO CHALLENGE YOURSELF

Generally, if you make an exercise or a workout harder for yourself to complete, it is going to be more beneficial for you. There are three things you can do to make the workouts more challenging.

1. INCREASE THE DIFFICULTY

Once you become confident and competent with an exercise and are finding that you are able to perform it easily, it is time to change it up and make it harder for yourself. You can make the exercise harder in two ways.

Firstly, you can slow down the tempo of the exercise. For example, perform a push-up more slowly, taking five seconds to lower your chest to the floor each time before pushing yourself back up.

Secondly, you can substitute the exercise for a more difficult version. For example, if you are breezing through your regular push-ups, you could try doing a clap push-up instead. Other examples of this type of progression include substituting a squat for a squat jump, a lunge for a jumping lunge, a body-weight row for a pull-up, a sprawl for a burpee, or a pike push-up for a handstand push-up.

2. INCREASE THE REPS

As you become better at doing these exercises you will find that you are able to do more and more reps with the same amount of effort or within the same timeframe. Push yourself to do more reps in an allocated time or just up the number of reps required to complete the workout.

3. DECREASE THE REST

As your muscular endurance and cardiovascular fitness improve you may find that you are not as short of breath as you were and you are able to take shorter breaks between exercises. Generally, the shorter the rest intervals you take, the more elevated your heart rate will remain, increasing your cardiovascular fitness and helping you to burn more fat.

CONCENTRIC AND ECCENTRIC CONTRACTIONS

To get the greatest benefit from these exercises, you need to know about the concentric and eccentric contraction of your muscles. A concentric contraction occurs when the muscle shortens, while an eccentric contraction occurs when it elongates. For example, during a squat, the concentric contraction of your quadriceps muscle occurs when you're going from the squat position to upright, while the eccentric contraction happens when you're lowering from standing into the squat. Likewise, the concentric contraction of your pectoral muscles in a push-up occurs when you are pushing back up, and the eccentric when you are lowering yourself down. And, as in the diagram of someone doing a guns workout (see following page), the concentric contraction occurs when you lift and pull the weight towards your body (the muscle is getting shorter) and the eccentric when the weight is lowered (the muscle elongates).

The way to get the most benefit from these exercises is to always make the eccentric contraction nice and slow and controlled, and the concentric fast and explosive. Think about controlling your descent into a squat or push-up, then releasing it with force and power. You will gain more benefit from a controlled eccentric contraction (taking anywhere from two to five seconds) than just relaxing and letting the resistance rapidly elongate the muscle.

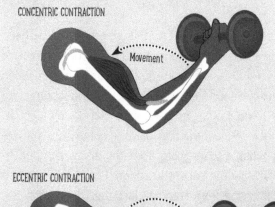

CONCENTRIC CONTRACTION

Movement

ECCENTRIC CONTRACTION

Movement

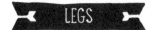

SQUATS

Stand with your feet shoulder width apart, with your weight through your heels.

Bend your knees and squat down. Your knees will go forward a bit but should not be in front of your toes. (A good indicator of correct technique is that you can see your toes over your knees the whole time — if you can't see your toes this means that you are loading up your knees with too much weight and can cause injury.) Keep your weight in your heels. Bend your knees until your thighs are parallel (or just below parallel) to the ground, then stand back up, keeping your weight in your heels.

Note: it doesn't matter what you do with your arms for this exercise, as long as you are not using them to push yourself up off your thighs. Have them loose at your sides, stretched out in front of you, clasped in front of your chest, or on your hips.

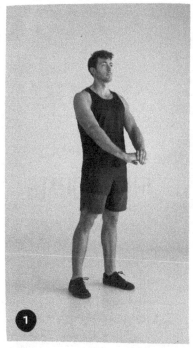
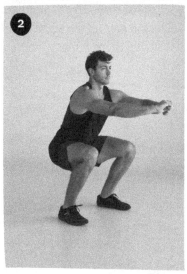

JUMP SQUATS

Make squats a bit harder by jumping as high as you can from your squat position. Land with bent knees back in the squat position, making sure your weight is still through your heels as you squat down. Try to jump and land back in the squat in one smooth movement.

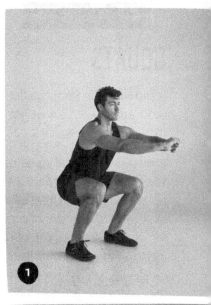

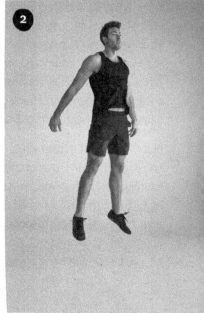

LUNGES

From standing upright, take a big step forward with one leg and bend your front knee until your thigh is parallel with the ground, moving your weight on to your front foot. Drop your back knee so that it is as close to the ground as possible but not touching it. Push back off your front foot to stand up again. Then repeat with your other leg. Maintain an upright chest and torso with your hips pushed forward the entire time — don't bend forward at the hips.

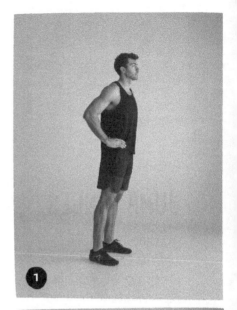

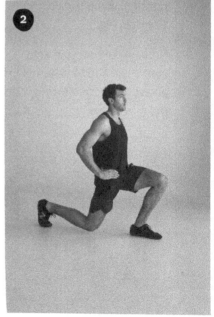

If you have room, walk forward in this fashion, going from lunge to lunge, alternating the leading leg. Essentially you'll be walking with giant steps.

You can just keep your arms by your sides or on your hips, but if you want to work your core more hold your arms above your head, with your hands loosely laced together.

JUMP LUNGES

From the lunge position, jump up and switch legs in the air, landing with the other leg forward into the lunge position. Jump back to the alternate leg.

Note: make sure your keep your chest and torso upright and core engaged throughout the movement.

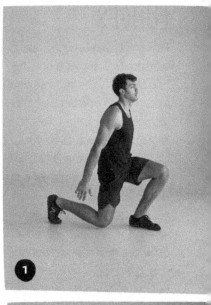

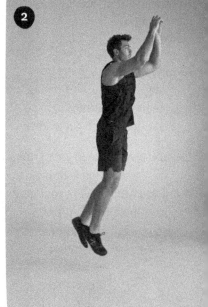

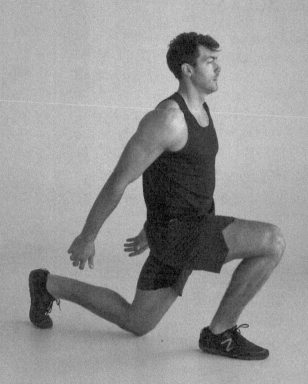

FROG ROCKS

Stand with your feet wider than hip width apart. Lean forward and place your elbows inside your knees, with your knees softly bent. Keep your hands out in front of you, with your fingers linked together.

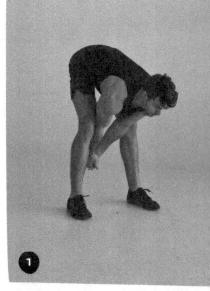

Rock down into a low squat position, then straighten your legs completely while still bending over (back to how you started). Your elbows will remain glued to the inside of your knees the entire time.

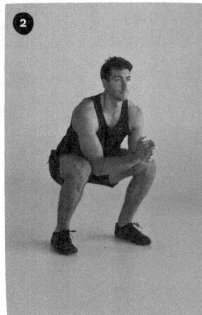

Note: this exercise can be done as quick or slow as you like.

HIP RAISES

Lie on your back with your knees bent, your legs forming a 90-degree angle, and your feet hip width apart. Place your hands by your sides or across your chest.

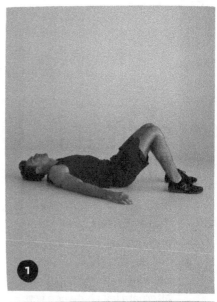

Lift your hips as high off the ground as they can go, engaging your gluteus muscles (your butt) as you go. Keep your body nice and straight from your knees down to your chest, with your hips lifting upwards. Lower to the ground, and repeat.

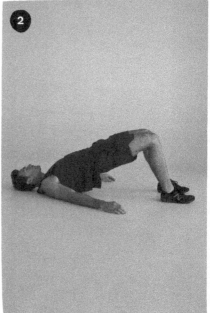

SINGLE-LEG HIP RAISES

Do the same thing as with the regular hip raises (see previous page), but elevate one leg straight in the air, keeping your thighs parallel. Alternate legs between sets.

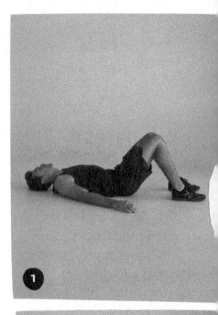

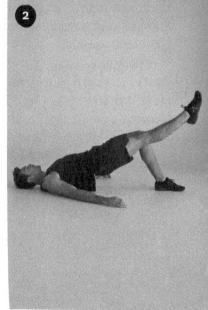

PISTOL SQUATS

Stand on one leg, with the other leg straightened out in front of you and your foot slightly off the ground. Hold your arms out in front of you.

Drop down into a one-legged squat as low as you can, holding your lifted leg and arms out in front of you off the ground. Stand back up again.

Make sure your movements are slow and controlled, keeping your back straight, with your chest as upright as possible throughout the squat.

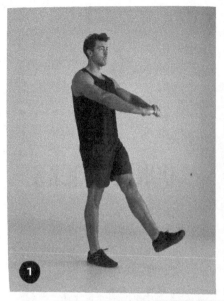

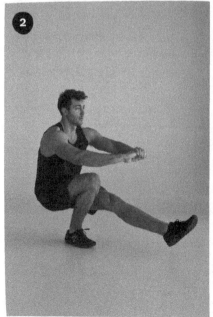

DONKEY KICKS

Get on to your hands and knees, with your knees close together and your hands under your shoulders.

Kick both your feet up towards your bottom at the same time, and jump them down to one side. Kick and jump back to the other side. Continue jumping side to side like this as if jumping over an imaginary fence.

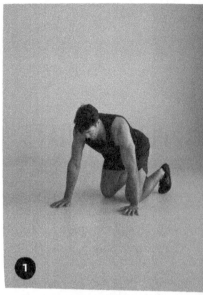

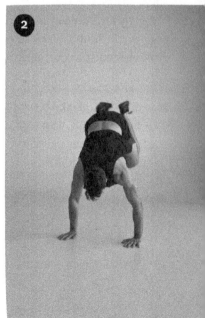

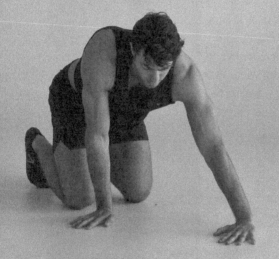

PUSH-UPS

Start on your hands and feet, or on your hands and knees if that's too difficult, with your body in a straight line, your hands a bit wider than your shoulders, fingers facing forward, and your feet slightly apart.

Slowly lower your body down until your chest touches the ground, or your chin almost touches the ground, then push back up again.

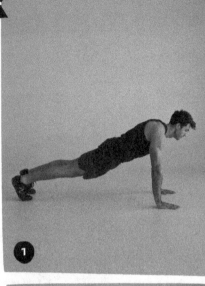

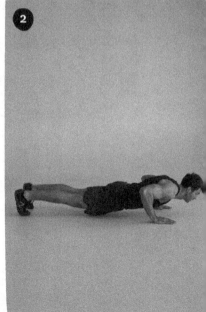

DIAMOND PUSH-UPS

Use the same technique as the push-ups (see opposite page), but place your hands close together under your sternum (the middle of your chest), with your fingers facing inwards and your thumbs touching, so your hands form a diamond directly under your chest.

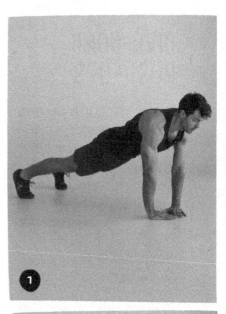

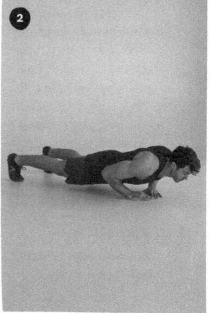

DIVE-BOMB PUSH-UPS

Start on your hands and feet, with your hands forward of your head and slightly wider than your shoulders. Place your feet wider than shoulder width apart, with your legs straight and bottom up, and look back at your feet. Try to imagine you're forming a capital A with your body.

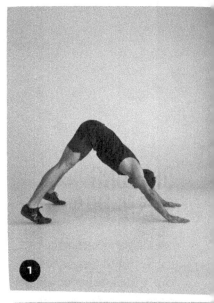

Drop and slide forward, bending your elbows into a push-up position. Lead with your head, followed by your chest, then straighten your arms, lifting your head and arching your back. Your hips will follow through — keep them just off the ground. Reverse the movement back to that A shape, with your bottom raised and legs straight. If you're familiar with yoga, this is similar to going from a downward dog to a cobra position and back again.

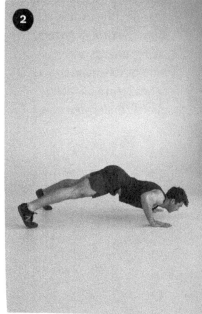

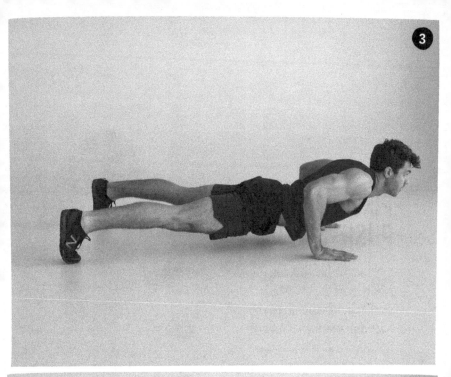

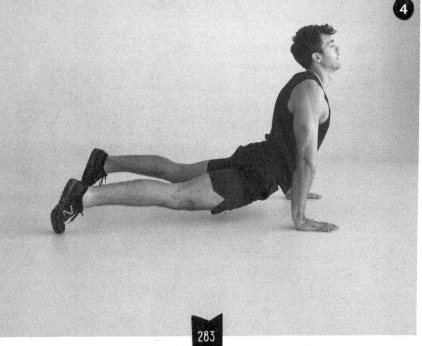

PIKE PUSH-UPS

Start in the same A-shape position as the dive-bomb push-up. Rise up on to your toes and bend your elbows until your head is just touching the ground then push back up to straight arms, always looking back at your feet.

Note: this is like a shoulder push-up — your elbows should bend outwards, so have your fingers pointing slightly inwards to make that happen.

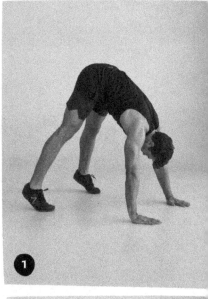

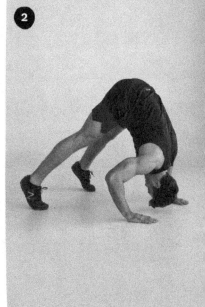

CLAP PUSH-UPS

Do a regular push-up (see page 280) but explode upwards, so that your momentum lifts your body off the ground. Clap your hands under your chest before putting them back down and doing the next push-up.

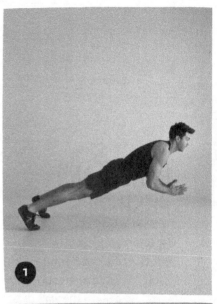

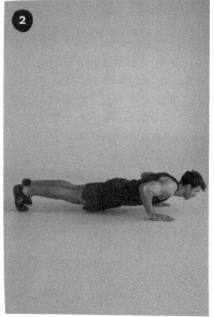

HANDSTAND PUSH-UPS

Go into a handstand
position, with your hands
shoulder width apart and
your feet against the wall.
Keep your fingers pointing
straight towards the wall.

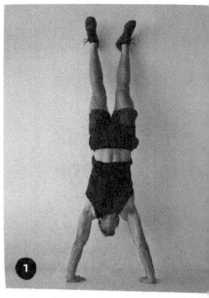

Slowly bend your elbows to
lower your head towards the
ground, then straighten your
arms, pushing your body
back up again. Remember
to breathe.

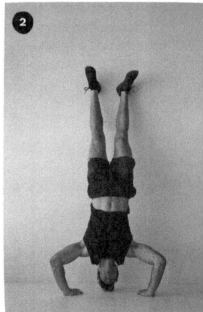

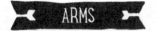
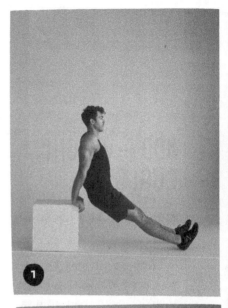

DIPS

Place a chair or something of a similar height behind you. Squat down so your hands are flat on the structure, fingers facing forward, and your arms straight. Straighten your legs out in front of you, with your feet hip width apart.

Bend your elbows out behind you to a 90-degree angle, lowering your bottom. Push back up to straight arms.

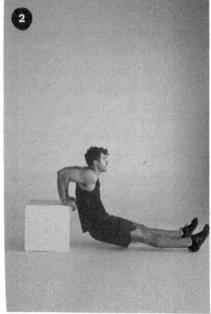

BODY-WEIGHT CURLS

You will need a low bar for this one.

Get your body under the bar, gripping it with your hands shoulder width apart, using an under grip, with your palms facing towards you and your fingers over the top. Keeping your legs straight, pull your chest up towards the bar. Lower back down to straight arms.

Keep your body, from head to toe, straight and rigid the whole time, with your core engaged.

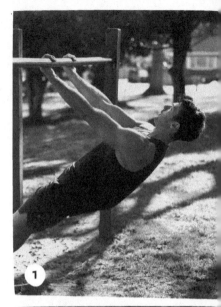

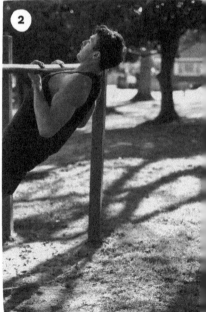

CHIN-UPS

This time you will need a higher bar.

Hang off the bar with your hands shoulder width apart, using an under grip (palms facing you). Pull yourself up so your chin is above the bar, engaging your core so you don't swing back and forth. Lower yourself back down in a controlled fashion.

Keep your body nice and straight — it should be your arms doing the work.

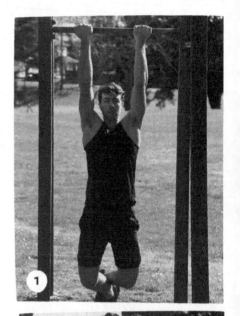

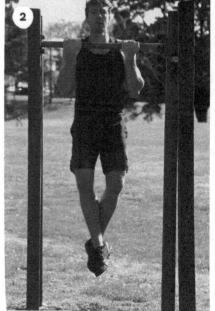

PULL-UPS

This is the same as a chin-up (see previous page), but use an over grip instead, with your palms facing away from you. Pull yourself up so your chin is above the bar.

This might seem like the same exercise as the chin-up, but it uses and works slightly different muscles because of the different hand position. Your biceps are comprised of two heads (essentially two different muscles, hence the name biceps, bi meaning two), and one lies under the other. Pull-ups work one of these muscles more, and chin-ups work the other one more.

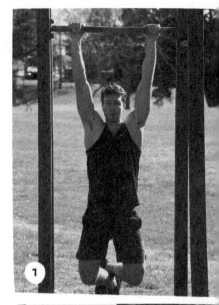

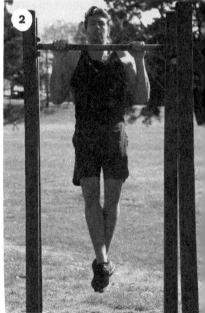

TRICEP EXTENSIONS

Once again you will need a low bar.

Lean forward and place your hands on the bar, with your arms straight. Your toes should be on the ground with your feet hip width apart. Engage your core to keep your body rigid and straight.

Bending at the elbows, lower your body down towards the ground, keeping your elbows pointing towards the ground and your body rigid. Straighten your arms again.

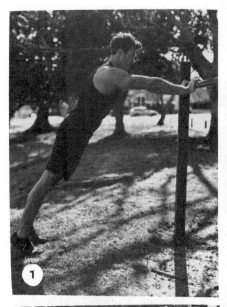

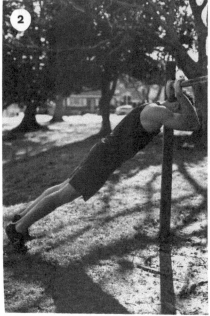

TRICEP PUSH-UPS

Start on your hands and feet, or on your hands and knees if that's too difficult, with your body in a straight line, your hands shoulder width apart and down in line with the bottom of your chest. Your fingers should be facing forward and your feet slightly apart. This is essentially the same starting position as a regular push-up but with your hands closer together and lower down your body.

Slowly lower your body down to the ground into a push-up position, but as you bend your arms bring your elbows backwards so that your elbows graze the sides of your body and you engage your triceps. Push back up again.

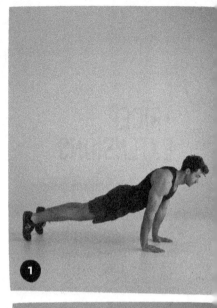

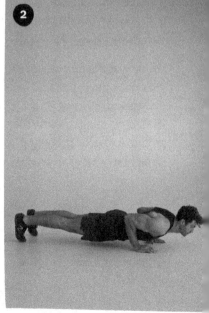

CYCLE CRUNCHES

Lie on your back on the floor with your knees bent, your hands behind your head and your core engaged.

Extended one of your legs out straight, without touching your foot to the ground. Touch your opposite elbow to your bent knee, twisting as much as possible and keeping your shoulders off the ground. Bring that straight leg back to bent and extend the other, twisting and crunching your abdominals.

Alternate your legs in a cycling action: elbow to knee, elbow to knee.

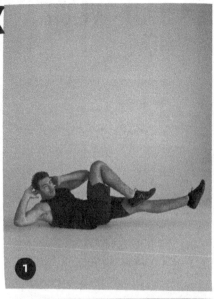

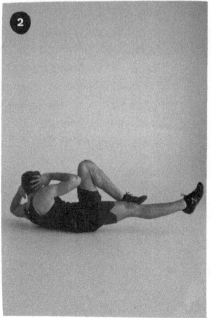

BODY-WEIGHT ROW

This exercise uses a low bar again.

Get your body under the bar, gripping it with an over grip (palms facing away from you) and your hands a bit wider than shoulder width apart. Place your heels on the ground, feet hip width apart. Your body should be straight and rigid, engaging your core throughout.

Pull your chest up to the bar, squeezing your shoulder blades together behind you. (Think about opening up your chest and pulling your shoulder blades together at the back.) Lower yourself back down in a slow and controlled fashion.

Your shoulders should be off the ground at the lowest extension, not lying on the ground.

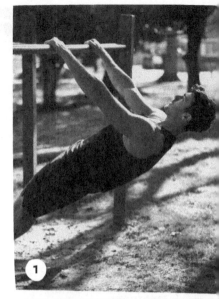

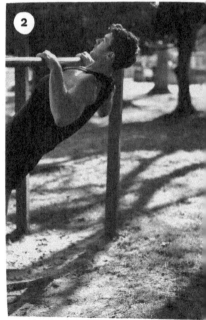

PLANK

Lie face down on your elbows and toes, with your elbows under your shoulders and your hands laced together. Keep your body as straight, still and rigid as possible, with your core engaged. Hold this position for as long as specified in the workout.

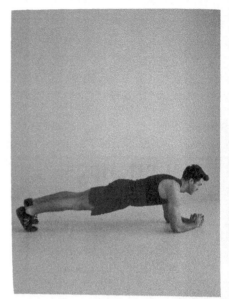

SUPERMAN

Lie on the floor on your stomach with your arms extended in front of you and your legs straight out behind you, as long as they can be, like Superman flying. Lift your arms and legs off the ground at same time and hold this position for as long as specified in the workout, leaving only your torso on the ground.

Don't tip your neck back; keep your neck and head relaxed as if you are looking forward to where you are flying.

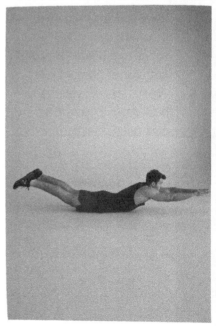

V SIT-UPS

Lie down flat on your back on the floor, with your arms stretched out above your head and your legs out straight.

Raise your legs and torso at same time to touch your hands to your feet, keeping both halves of your body straight. Unfold your body back down to lying in a controlled fashion.

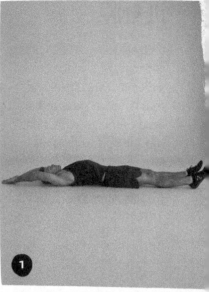

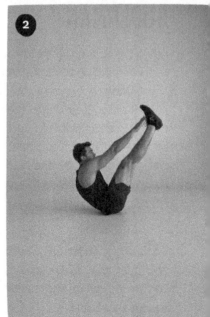

FLUTTER KICKS

Lie on your back with your hands by your sides (or under your bottom, to ease any strain on your lower back). Raise your feet a few centimetres off the ground and kick them as if swimming. Both legs should be off the ground at once, with your head elevated so you are looking at your feet.

Keep your legs nice and straight, and use small, controlled movements.

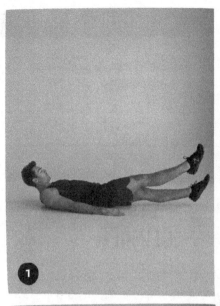

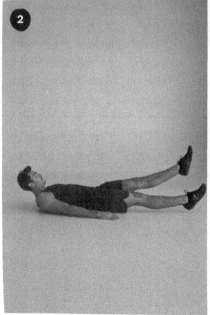

This is where you can really add some cardio to your workout, by doing these exercises at pace with few rest breaks.

MOUNTAIN CLIMBER

Start off in push-up position. Jump one leg forward into a low lunge position under your chest, keeping the other leg straight (similar to the body position of a sprinter about to take off). Push your hips up to swap feet, jumping the other foot forward under your body and extending the first leg out straight. Repeat this as fast as you can, switching legs as you jump.

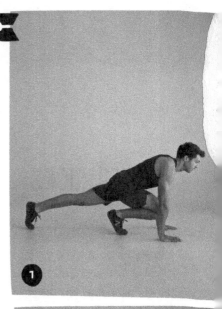

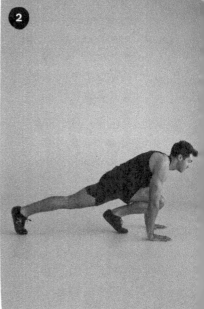

LATERAL MOUNTAIN CLIMBER

Starting in push-up position again, pull one knee up to touch your elbow on the outside of your body and extend it back out straight. Repeat as fast as you can, alternating legs.

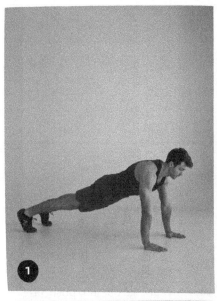

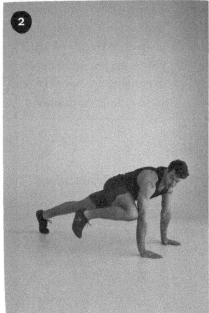

SPRAWLS

From standing, place your hands on the floor, jump your legs out into push-up position, then jump them back in to your chest, and jump up in the air. (If you have knee problems or are uncomfortable jumping, just go to a standing position.)

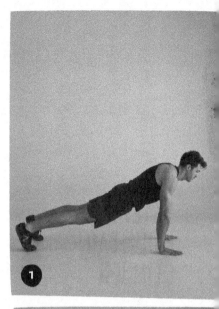

1

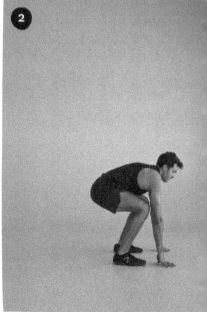

2

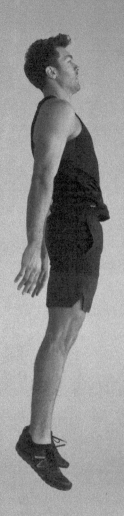

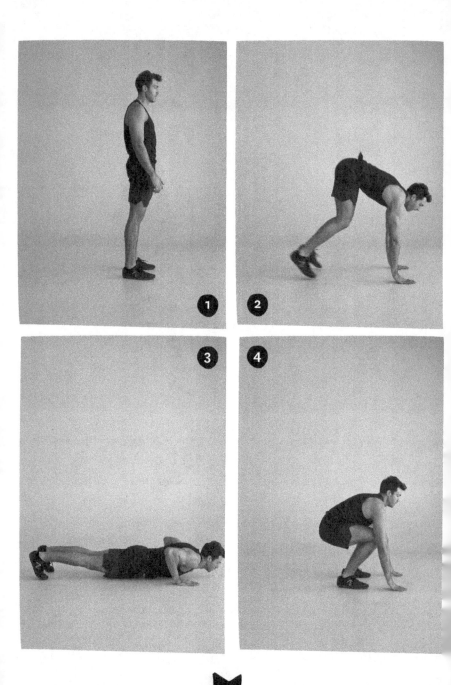

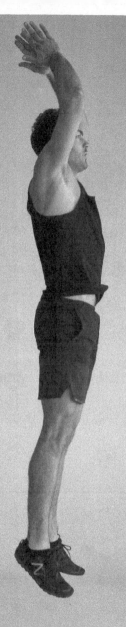

BURPEES

This is the best full-body exercise you can do, just using your body weight.

Use the same technique as for sprawls (see previous pages), but do a push-up at the bottom (when in the high plank position, push down to the ground and up again) and jump in the air when you come up. I like to clap my hands high above my head when I jump, as this makes me jump higher and more upright.

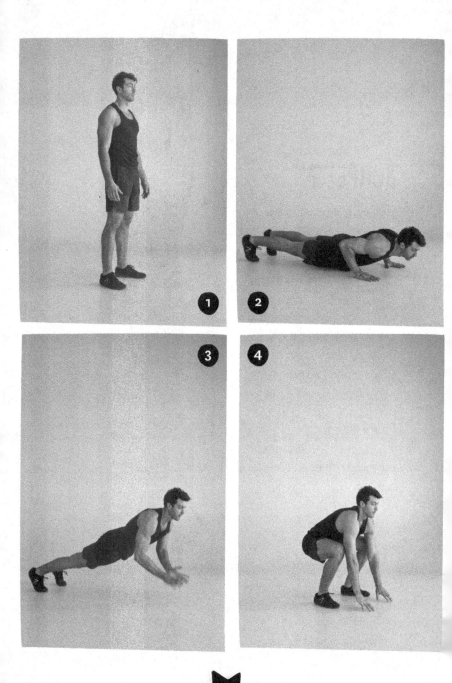

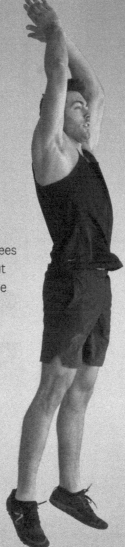

CLAP BURPEES

Do the same as the burpees on the previous pages but with a clap push-up in the middle. Clap your hands together when you jump up also.

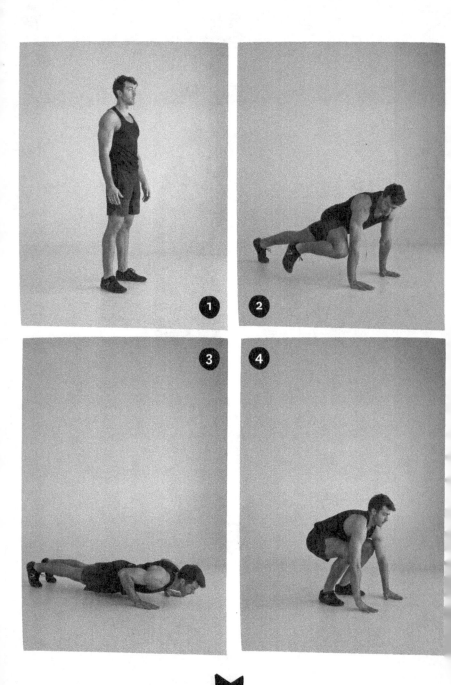

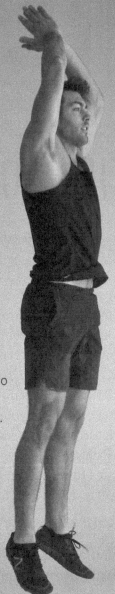

LATERAL MOUNTAIN-CLIMBER BURPEES

From standing, drop down to your hands and feet. Perform one lateral mountain-climber (see page 299) on each side, do a push-up, then a squat jump back up to standing.

20. THE WORKOUTS

· · · · · · · · · · · · · · ·

Cool, now that you know the exercises, it's time to put them together into structured workouts. In the following pages you will learn some of the best and most effective routines to combine the exercises into fun, challenging, full-body workouts. Once you have given these routines a go and got the hang of them, you can then become your own trainer and tailor your workouts to suit your goals. You can substitute a leg exercise for an arm exercise here, or change some press-ups for squats there because you want to work your legs. Whatever you do, just remember to go hard! Pain is temporary; results are long term.

All of these workouts will increase your cardio fitness, muscular endurance, strength and flexibility. They are all functional high-intensity interval training workouts.

EMOM stands for Every Minute On the Minute. Doing a short EMOM workout can be a great warm-up to a longer workout, or you can combine multiple EMOMs for a complete workout.

The basic template is this: you perform X number of reps (repetitions) of a specific exercise (your 'minute exercise') on every minute (each time the clock shows :00), then complete as many reps as possible of another exercise (your 'scoring exercise') in the remaining time left in that minute. You will do this for a set number of minutes in total.

So, using EMOM 1 on the next page as an example, start the timer and do 10 burpees, then start doing lunge jumps and count them until the timer gets to 1 minute — ideally use a stopwatch or an app on your phone that can beep every minute. Once the minute is up, you then do another 10 burpees before returning to your lunge jumps, keeping count of them again, for the remainder of that minute. Continue doing this for 10 minutes in total.

Your score is how many lunge jumps you performed in total over the 10 minutes. You will find that the further through the workout you get, the more fatigued you become and the minute exercise (your burpees) will take longer to complete; this leaves less time for the scoring exercises (your lunge jumps). You can use the score to track your fitness progression.

EMOM 1

Target muscle groups: Legs / full body
Time: 10 minutes
Minute exercise: 10 burpees
Scoring exercise: Lunge jumps (or lunges)

EMOM 2

Target muscle groups: Chest / full body
Time: 5 minutes
Minute exercise: 10 burpees
Scoring exercise: Push-ups

EMOM 3

Target muscle groups: Abs / full body
Time: 10 minutes
Minute exercise: 20 lateral mountain climbers
Scoring exercise: V sit-ups

CIRCUITS

The following circuits involve a set number of reps or amount of time on each exercise. The idea with this type of circuit is to complete all of the exercises in quick succession, resting as little as possible in between. If you feel the need to rest, try to do so in between rounds, and aim for 30 seconds to 1 minute. Feel free to change the exercises round and mix it up a bit to work different parts of your body. Time yourself to track your progress.

CIRCUIT 1

Target muscle groups: Full body
Time: As fast as possible
Rounds: Complete 3 full rounds

→ 50 mountain climbers
→ 40 lunge jumps (or lunges)
→ 30 push-ups
→ 20 donkey kicks
→ 10 burpees or sprawls
→ 20 pike push-ups
→ 30 squat jumps (or squats)
→ 40 frog rocks
→ 50 lateral mountain climbers

CIRCUIT 2

Target muscle groups: Abs and back
Time: As fast as possible
Rounds: Complete 3 full rounds

→ 50-second plank
→ 40 flutter kicks (2 kicks = 1 rep)
→ 30 cycle crunches (each side = 1 rep)
→ 20 V sit-ups
→ 1-minute superman hold
→ 20 V sit-ups
→ 30 cycle crunches (each side = 1 rep)
→ 40 flutter kicks (2 kicks = 1 rep)
→ 50-second plank

CIRCUIT 3

Target muscle groups: Full body

Time: As fast as possible

Rounds: Complete 1 full round

- → 100 flutter kicks (2 kicks = 1 rep)
- → 90 mountain climbers
- → 80 squat jumps (or squats)
- → 70 cycle crunches (each side = 1 rep)
- → 60 tricep dips
- → 50 lunge jumps (or lunges)
- → 40 donkey kicks
- → 30 V sit-ups
- → 20 diamond push-ups
- → 10 burpees
- → 5 handstand push-ups (or pike push-ups)
- → 10 burpees
- → 20 diamond push-ups
- → 30 V sit-ups
- → 40 donkey kicks
- → 50 lunge jumps (or lunges)
- → 60 tricep dips
- → 70 cycle crunches (each side = 1 rep)
- → 80 squat jumps (or squats)
- → 90 mountain climbers
- → 100 flutter kicks (2 kicks = 1 rep)

AMRAP WORKOUTS

AMRAP stands for As Many Rounds As Possible. This means that in a set amount of time you are to complete as many rounds of a circuit as possible. So, using AMRAP 1 below as an example, you complete 5 burpees, then 5 pull-ups, then 5 squat jumps, then 5 V sit-ups, then 5 dive-bomb push-ups – and all this is 1 round. Do as many rounds as you can in 15 minutes, resting as little as possible in between rounds.

AMRAP 1

Target muscle groups: Full body
Time: 15 minutes
Rounds: As many as possible
- → 5 burpees (or sprawls)
- → 5 pull-ups (or body-weight rows)
- → 5 squat jumps (or squats)
- → 5 V sit-ups
- → 5 dive-bomb push-ups

AMRAP 2

Target muscle groups: Full body
Time: 10 minutes
Rounds: As many as possible
- → 5 chin-ups (or body-weight curls)
- → 6 lunge jumps (or lunges)
- → 7 diamond push-ups
- → 8 donkey kicks
- → 9 sprawls
- → 10 dips

AMRAP 3

Target muscle groups: Abs and legs
Time: 15 minutes

Rounds: As many as possible
- → 10 V sit-ups
- → 20 frog rocks
- → 30 cycle crunches (each side = 1 rep)
- → 40 hip raises (or 20 single-leg raises on each side)
- → 50 flutter kicks (2 kicks = 1 rep)

DEVIL WORKOUTS

I call these Devil Workouts because they require you to perform 6 reps of 6 exercises 6 times over, and 666 is supposedly the Devil's number! It's pretty straightforward — you just complete the 6 rounds of 6 reps of each exercise as fast as you can, resting as little as possible in between each round.

DEVIL 1
Target muscle groups: Full body
Time: As fast as possible
Rounds: 6
- → 6 push-ups
- → 6 donkey kicks on each side (12 jumps in total)
- → 6 tricep extensions
- → 6 burpees
- → 6 body-weight rows
- → 6 squat jumps

DEVIL 2
Target muscle groups: Full body (advanced)

Time: As fast as possible

Rounds: 6

- → 6 dive-bomb push-ups
- → 6 lunge jumps on each leg (12 jumps in total)
- → 6 handstand push-ups (or pike push-ups)
- → 6 lateral mountain climber burpees
- → 6 chin-ups
- → 6 pistol squats (3 on each leg)

DEVIL 3

Target muscle groups: Legs

Time: As fast as possible

Rounds: 6

- → 6 squat jumps
- → 6 lunge jumps on each leg (12 jumps in total)
- → 6 frog rocks
- → 6 mountain climbers on each leg (12 jumps in total)
- → 6 donkey kicks on each side (12 jumps in total)
- → 6 single-leg hip raises on each leg (12 jumps in total)

TABATA

Tabata training is a widely used form of high-intensity interval training (HIIT). Before I explain the workout, I'm going to give a brief history of Tabata, because I think it's quite interesting.

The term Tabata comes from the guy who invented it, Dr Izumi Tabata, a Japanese scientist from the National Institute of Fitness and Sports in Tokyo. Dr

Tabata performed an experiment with two groups of Olympic speed skaters, where the first group trained at a moderate intensity for a long duration while the second group trained at a high intensity for only 4 minutes a day (consisting of 20 seconds of exercise followed by 10 seconds of rest repeated eight times). What Dr Tabata found was that the first group improved their aerobic system (cardiovascular fitness) but showed little or no results for their anaerobic system (muscular strength, speed and power). The second group showed an even greater improvement in their aerobic system *and* improved their anaerobic system significantly. In conclusion, Dr Tabata proved that high-intensity interval training has a greater impact on both the aerobic and anaerobic systems.

With Tabata training, you pair two exercises up and work them both in the same 4-minute Tabata set. So, using Tabata 1 opposite as an example, you perform 20 seconds of squat jumps at maximum effort, then rest for 10 seconds, then do 20 seconds of donkey kicks at maximum effort, then rest for 10 seconds before starting back on another 20 seconds of squat jumps and so forth. This is repeated until you have done a total of four lots of squat jumps and four lots of donkey kicks, which will take you 4 minutes. I'd suggest downloading a Tabata app on your phone that will beep at the 20-second and 10-second intervals — there are plenty of free ones available.

TABATA 1

Target muscle groups: Legs / full body

Time: 4 minutes in total

Rounds: 4

- → 20 seconds squat jumps
- → 10 seconds rest
- → 20 seconds donkey kicks
- → 10 seconds rest

TABATA 2

Target muscle groups: Chest / full body

Time: 4 minutes in total

Rounds: 4

- → 20 seconds burpees
- → 10 seconds rest
- → 20 seconds push-ups
- → 10 seconds rest

TABATA 3

Target muscle groups: Abs

Time: 4 minutes in total

Rounds: 4

- → 20 seconds cycle crunches
- → 10 seconds rest
- → 20 seconds V sit-ups
- → 10 seconds rest

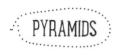
PYRAMIDS

There are many different variations of Pyramid-type workouts. Here are three of my favourites.

FULL PYRAMIDS

This pyramid workout involves performing a total of 19 rounds with first ascending then descending numbers of reps and exercises. The idea is to charge through the rounds with as little rest as possible in between.

Using the example on pages 320–321, you will start off with 1 burpee in Round 1, and then go straight on to Round 2 to perform 1 burpee and 2 V sit-ups. Round 3 will be 1 Burpee, 2 V sit-ups and 3 pull-ups. At Round 10 you will reach the top of the pyramid; once you've completed your 10 lateral mountain-climber burpees, you will begin to drop one exercise each round until you perform your last burpee in Round 19.

Target muscle groups: Full body
Time: As fast as possible
See table over page.

STANDARD PYRAMID

This pyramid workout involves performing each exercise for increasing and then decreasing numbers of reps. In the workout below, for example, you will perform 2 reps of each exercise, then 4 reps of each, then 6 reps, and so on.

Target muscle groups: Full body
Time: As fast as possible
Reps: 2 – 4 – 6 – 8 – 10 – 12 – 10 – 8 – 6 – 4 – 2

Exercises:

- → Burpees
- → Squat jumps
- → Lateral mountain climbers
- → Dive-bomb push-ups
- → V sit-ups

ACCUMULATIVE PYRAMID

This pyramid workout involves performing 1 rep of each exercise, then 2 reps, then 3 reps, and so on. Continue for a designated amount of time, pushing yourself to reach the highest number of reps that you can in that amount of time.

Target muscle groups: Full body

Time: 20 minutes

Rounds and reps: As many as possible

Exercises:

- → Squat jumps (or squats)
- → Dive-bomb push-ups
- → Chin-ups
- → Lunge jumps
- → Pike push-ups (or handstand push-ups)
- → Clap burpees
- → Tricep extensions

300S

The 300 workout became popular a few years ago when the movie 300 was released. The idea is that the actors on the movie got in great shape by doing a 300 workout,

FULL PYRAMID

NUMBER OF REPS									
10									
9									FR
8								PUSH	PUSH
7							SJ	SJ	SJ
6						LMC	LMC	LMC	LMC
5					DBPU	DBPU	DBPU	DBPU	DBPU
4				LJ	LJ	LJ	LJ	LJ	LJ
3			PULL	PULL	PULL	PULL	PULL	PULL	PULL
2		VSU	VSU	VSU	VSU	VSU	VSU	VSU	VSU
1	B	B	B	B	B	B	B	B	B
	1	2	3	4	5	6	7	8	9

ROUND NUMBER

KEY	
LMCB	Lateral mountain-climber burpees
FR	Frog rocks
PUSH	Push-ups
SJ	Squat jumps
LMC	Lateral mountain climbers
DBPU	Dive-bomb push-ups
LJ	Lunge jumps
PULL	Pull-ups
VSU	V sit-ups
B	Burpee

LMCB									
FR	FR								
PUSH	PUSH	PUSH							
SJ	SJ	SJ	SJ						
LMC	LMC	LMC	LMC	LMC					
DBPU	DBPU	DBPU	DBPU	DBPU	DBPU				
LJ	LJ	LJ	LJ	LJ	LJ	LJ			
PULL	PULL	PULL	PULL	PULL	PULL	PULL	PULL		
VSU	VSU	VSU	VSU	VSU	VSU	VSU	VSU	VSU	
B	B	B	B	B	B	B	B	B	B
10	11	12	13	14	15	16	17	18	19

which involved performing different numbers of reps of various exercises to a total of 300 reps.

The goal of these workouts is to complete the 300 total reps as quickly as you can. You can do the exercises in any order, and break up the rep count however you want, as long as you complete the amount of reps of each exercise — and, therefore, the total 300 reps. These workouts are a great way to track your progress.

CLASSIC 300
Target muscle groups: Full body
Time: As fast as possible

→ 25 pull-ups (or body-weight rows)
→ 50 squat jumps (or squats)
→ 50 push-ups
→ 50 lunge jumps (or lunges)
→ 50 V sit-ups (or cycle crunches)
→ 50 dips
→ 25 chin-ups (or body-weight curls)

LEG 300
Target muscle groups: Legs
Time: As fast as possible

→ 50 squat jumps
→ 50 donkey kicks
→ 50 mountain climbers
→ 50 lunge jumps
→ 50 hip raises (25 on each leg)
→ 50 frog rocks

ADVANCED 300

Target muscle groups: Full body

Time: As fast as possible

- → 25 lateral mountain-climber burpees
- → 50 dips
- → 50 lunge jumps
- → 25 clap push-ups
- → 25 pike push-ups
- → 50 squat jumps
- → 50 V sit-ups
- → 25 clap burpees

20/20S

20/20s use only two exercises. They involve going from 1 rep up to 20 reps of one exercise, while at the same time going from 20 reps of the other exercise down to 1 rep. So, using the Standard 20/20 below as an example, you would perform 1 frog rock and then 20 dips, then 2 frog rocks and 19 dips, and so on. You would keep going until you perform 20 frog rocks and 1 dip.

STANDARD 20/20

Target muscle groups: Legs / triceps

Time: As fast as possible

Reps: 1–20 and 20–1

Exercises:

- → Frog rocks
- → Dips

MODERATE 20/20

Target muscle groups: Legs / chest

Time: As fast as possible

Reps: 1–20 and 20–1

Exercises:

→ Squat jumps (or squats)

→ Push-ups

ADVANCED 20/20

Target muscle groups: Full body / shoulders

Time: As fast as possible

Reps: 1–20 and 20–1

Exercises:

→ Burpees

→ Pike push-ups

21. LACE UP YOUR SHOES
PUTTING THE WORKOUTS INTO ACTION

........•

If you want to, you can just incorporate these workouts into your normal weekly exercise routine in whatever way you see fit. However, if you are after a bit more structure and want to see some real fitness results, have a go at following this plan.

WEEKS 1 AND 2: TRIAL PERIOD

The first two weeks are a trial period. Start this period off by going through all of the individual exercises and trying them out. See how many reps you can do of each to gauge how difficult they are.

Next, you want to spend these two weeks trialling as many of the different workouts as you can. Aim for about 30-60 minutes of exercise per day — so that may mean anywhere between one and four different workouts a day, depending on which ones you do (some take far less time than others).

Don't push yourself too hard in these first two weeks, as the purpose is to familiarise yourself with the different workouts and how they make you feel. And listen to your body; if you're sore, then have a rest for a day or two, or do a workout that will work your muscles which aren't sore. This trial period will give you an idea of your base fitness level, which exercises and workout styles you enjoy, and which ones you find difficult.

EXAMPLE FIRST THREE WEEKS

WEEK	MONDAY	TUESDAY	WEDNESDAY	THURSDAY
1 TRIAL PERIOD	EMOM 1 TABATA 2	Circuit 1	EMOM 2 AMRAP 1	Rest Day
2 TRIAL PERIOD	Circuit 2 AMRAP 2	Standard 20/20 EMOM 3	AMRAP 3	EMOM 3 Devil 1
3 TESTING WORKOUTS	EMOM 2 Standard 20/20		Classic 300	

WEEK 3: TESTING

Now you want to take some baseline fitness measurements or times. For this you need to choose between three and five different workouts — these are going to become your testing workouts. Choose them based on how much you enjoy them, how much you want to challenge yourself, and how specific they are in helping you to reach your fitness goals.

Give these workouts your best shot, performing them with maximum effort, and record their respective fitness marker (this is your time, or number of rounds or reps).

You don't need to rush these testing workouts. There's no need to try to do them all on one day — although you can if you like. Otherwise, you can just use the whole week to complete them, making sure that you are adequately rested before doing each workout so

FRIDAY	SATURDAY	SUNDAY
Standard Pyramid	Rest Day	Classic 300
Full Pyramid	Circuit 3	Rest Day
Full Pyramid		

that you can give it your best effort. Record your results and keep them somewhere that you won't lose them so you can refer back to them.

WEEKS 4 TO 7: GET FIT AND GO HARD

Spend the next weeks basically just performing as many of the workouts on pages 308-324 as you can every week. The ideal is to do at least one workout every day, even if it's just a short, 10-minute AMRAP on a Sunday morning. If you take a couple of days off, then try to make up for it on subsequent days. Aim for 30-60 minutes of exercise per day, or an average of 5-7 hours per week.

Try to get friends to do the workouts with you, as this will help to motivate you and make the workouts more enjoyable.

WEEK 8: RE-TEST

This week you will perform those testing workouts that you did back in week three again. Just like last time, you are to go as hard as you can and perform to the best of your ability. Record your results and compare them to your results from a month ago. Hopefully you will see a vast improvement!

WEEK 9 AND BEYOND

Continue to cycle through weeks of workouts, testing yourself as often as you like to measure your improvements. Mix up the workouts, create your own and just have fun.

> ➤**TIP**: Remember, rest is as important as exercise. Listen to your body, and if your muscles are sore give them a rest. This is your body talking to you and telling you to slow down and let it repair. If you don't give your body time to repair and grow stronger, then you will never improve or reach your goals as quickly.

SECTION 3
OTHER IMPORTANT STUFF

22. GETTING YOUR HEAD TOGETHER
AND KEEPING IT THAT WAY

．．．．．．．．．．．．．．．．

So, now you've read about how to nourish your body with the best possible nutrition, and how to use that as fuel to create and maintain your healthiest body through optimal exercise. Start putting this into practice, if you haven't already, and you will begin to feel amazing.

And that's what it's all about, really, isn't it? There's no point in making diet and lifestyle changes if they don't make you feel any better. We all want to feel happy, upbeat, positive, confident and healthy. And I bet that by thinking about what you eat and how you exercise you are starting to feel the benefits already.

But, before you run off thinking you're a changed person armed with everything you need to get healthy, lose weight, gain energy and so on, I think there is one major aspect of overall health and wellbeing that is sometimes overlooked; in my opinion, this is by far the most important part. I'm referring to your mental health. Your brain. The most important organ in your body. The brain allows us to think and feel, and enables us to have memories and emotions — all the things that make us human. And, when your brain isn't functioning optimally, the rest of your body won't be either.

Good mental health is paramount for a successful and satisfying life. It doesn't matter if you have surrounded yourself with possessions, or have some high-level job with a fancy title, or have a bangin' body if you're not happy with yourself and your life. Owning a bunch of things — and owing money on them — might be causing you stress, your job might be giving you sleepless nights, and the pressure to look good might be doing your head in. A lot of people think they will find happiness in possessions, jobs or social status — and often these things can give short-term happiness. Others might see happiness as a goal they will reach when they retire to a life of comfort.

But happiness is a mental state, it's a feeling, it is subjective and it cannot be bought. This eternal search for 'happiness' can consume some people, many of whom overlook the fact that when you're mentally healthy it doesn't matter what you have because you will most probably be happy anyway.

As mentioned earlier, I believe eating paleo and getting regular exercise can have huge mental-health benefits; indeed, all three (nutrition, exercise and mental health) are hugely interrelated and dependent on one another. But there are a few other things that I think are important to take care of to ensure you are feeling as good as possible throughout your whole body, including your brain.

SLEEP

This is first on the list because I believe it's the most important — I know it certainly is for me. Today's fast-paced world seems to demand as many waking hours from us as we can give. It's almost fashionable to be working extremely hard and getting by with very little sleep — Barack Obama is said to sleep for only six hours a night, and Donald Trump reckons he only needs three or four (perhaps that explains a few things . . .). Having a decent sleep every night has come to be seen in many instances as a sign of weakness or laziness. However, I believe adequate sleep — by which I mean about eight hours a night — is absolutely vital for keeping your brain healthy and your mood stable.

I know that when I'm feeling down, having negative thoughts about a situation, or just generally struggling to get excited about something, approximately 90 per cent of the time it's because I haven't had enough sleep. And then, because I'm aware of this and know how my body works, I do something about it by making sure I get the sleep I need to feel happy and positive again.

SLEEP BENEFITS

Many important bodily functions occur while we are getting a decent sleep, and provide a range of benefits.

→ Your breathing stabilises and slows, giving your cardiovascular system a rest. Your heart rate also slows and your blood pressure and body temperature drop.

→ The blood supply to your muscles increases, and tissue growth and repair occur. This is when you build your muscle, and often you will sleep more deeply after strenuous, heavy lifting and strength exercise so that your muscles can repair and grow.

→ Sleep helps to regulate levels of hormones which play a role in our feelings of hunger and fullness. If you're sleep-deprived, you may feel the need to eat more, which can lead to weight gain.

→ Inadequate sleep can also be associated with increases in the secretion of insulin following eating, which affects the body's ability to process glucose and promotes fat storage.

→ Although scientists haven't yet worked out why or how, it appears sleep is vital for the formation of memories and for retaining learnt information.

→ Poor sleep leads to an increase in the production of the stress hormone cortisol (again, this is what can cause you to store fat and make it harder to lose weight), and is connected to low mood.

I try to get eight hours' sleep a night, but it's not always easy. I like to be up at 5.30am to be at the gym at 6am, so my goal every night is to be in bed by 9.30pm. However, this doesn't always happen. Sleep is so important to me that I'll put it ahead of exercise on my to-do list if I think I am getting behind. I'd rather skip a workout and sleep in a bit to restore my sleep balance, because I know it will make me function better and feel more upbeat and positive.

Some people don't need as much sleep while others need a bit more — the American National Sleep Foundation says adults aged 24-60 need between seven and nine hours a night. But some scientific studies show that if you get less than seven hours a night on a regular basis, you are at higher risk of developing obesity, Type 2 diabetes and cardiovascular disease.

I find my exercise regime also helps a lot with my sleep. On the days that I exercise (which is pretty much every day, actually) I find I sleep better. I get to sleep more quickly and I wake up less in the night. Diet plays a role in this too — since I avoid coffee after 3pm there is very little caffeine in my system when I am trying to get to sleep, and because I don't eat refined sugar I am not being kept awake by sugar rushes either. (If you're not drinking coffee in the evenings but still have trouble getting drowsy, think about what else you might be eating or drinking which contains caffeine. Even dark chocolate can keep you awake if you're sensitive to caffeine. And, remember, green tea still contains caffeine.)

I usually don't have any trouble getting off to sleep, and I think this is predominantly because I tire myself out during the day both physically (with exercise) and mentally (with work). I do also try to avoid using screens — things like computers, phones and tablets — for half an hour before shutting my eyes. Think you won't survive? Try reading a book. I find books very effective at chilling me out, taking my mind off work and other daily stresses, and generally making me start to nod off. And if that's what you're using my book for then I don't mind. If that's what it can help you with, I'm happy!

I also don't exercise within an hour of wanting to go to sleep. While regular exercise helps me to feel sleepy by the end of the day and to stay asleep, it takes a while for your body to wind down after the exercise 'high' and be ready for sleep. Try to time your exercise sessions for when you can enjoy the sense of energy and alertness they provide afterwards — not when you are trying to relax and get to sleep.

If you need help to unwind, herbal teas can help. Chamomile tea is good, and you can also buy special herbal sleep blends.

RELAXATION AND STRESS MANAGEMENT

In order to enjoy good-quality sleep and all-round wellbeing it's really important to keep your stress levels down. Life is busy, I know, and work and social commitments can really stack up. That's why it's so important to find ways to manage your stress and take time out to relax in a way that suits you and your lifestyle.

Basically, the sensation of stress, caused by need or urgency, means your body calls on its fight-or-flight response, releasing hormones including cortisol and adrenalin into the blood. A little bit of this can be good, as it encourages your body and brain to find a solution to the stress challenge, but if your body goes on being swamped by these hormones it puts your entire system at risk. One of the other things your body does in response to stress hormones is store body fat, especially in that critical visceral region around your tummy and organs.

For me, exercise is the key to keeping my stress levels manageable — that and finding the balance between enough coffee and too much coffee (see opposite page)! But seriously, I know that a certain degree of stress can be beneficial for me, in terms of motivating me to perform at work or in a sporting situation. However, too much stress, for too long, is counterproductive and has negative effects, both in the short and long term, on your physical health. Stop being a hero about how much stress you're feeling and get it under control, for your health's sake.

EXERCISE

Exercising gives me energy and makes me feel happy. As I've discussed earlier, it releases endorphins, which make you feel good, plus gets lots of oxygen into your blood and pumped around your body. It's impossible to still feel grumpy and stressed after a good workout, a run or a swim. At the time you may feel too stressed, tired or stubborn to do anything, but just tie up those laces and get outside or on your bike or whatever. My dad always says that the hardest part about going for a run is getting your kit on. (He was referring, of course, to the mental barrier of convincing yourself to do it — not literally putting your kit on.)

COFFEE

As I discussed earlier, caffeine is that little double-edged sword so many of us have a love-hate relationship with. For me, I believe having a certain amount of it a day (in my case, no more than two coffees) helps to keep my mind sharp and better able to deal with stressful situations through quick thinking. However, put me in the same situation after having three or four coffees and I can feel quite uncomfortably stressed.

Think about your caffeine consumption and how it might be aiding or abetting your feelings of being stressed. Feeling shaky, nervous, anxious or overwhelmed might be more to do with your excessive coffee consumption than the situations you are having to deal with. Work out what is the optimum amount for you and don't be tempted to exceed it — it will make you feel worse, not better. And, again, keep in mind that coffee consumption = increased stress hormones = increased fat storage.

YOGA

You might have tried yoga as part of your exercise programme, to increase strength and flexibility, but it is also a powerful tool for relaxation and stress management. If you have done a yoga class before, you will have noticed how much emphasis is placed on breathing as you go through each set of movements and during the relaxation section at the end of the class. Learning how to use yoga breathing techniques in everyday situations can be a huge help when dealing with stress. It is a form of meditation, but a really easy one to learn and utilise in everyday life.

I sort of taught myself yoga. I'd been to a few yoga classes with friends before moving to Australia, but during my time at the mines I watched a lot of YouTube tutorials and read a few books, and taught myself the basics. I got into the habit of doing sun salutations in the mornings and some yoga moves after my workouts to cool down and stretch.

If you're just starting out, I'd recommend going to a class at your local gym or yoga centre. As with doing a fitness class, there's a nice energy to doing yoga in a room full of other people, plus you'll have the guidance (and sometimes firm hand!) of the instructor. It's useful to be able to follow the instructor's voice when you're still getting the hang of when to breathe in and when to breathe out, too.

Once you've learnt the basics, however, doing yoga is a bit like body-weight exercises: you can do it just about anywhere, any time you need a quick stress fix or a stretch to slow down, chill and relax. It's like a physical and mental workout all in one. I always come away from a yoga session feeling upbeat, clear-minded and like I've had a full-body massage and a spa bath.

In an ideal world where I didn't have a thousand and one other commitments, I would love to have time to do yoga at least three times a week. I'll keep working on that . . .

BREATHING TO RELAX

As I've mentioned above with yoga, thinking about your breathing can be a very effective way to relax and decrease stress. One type of breathing that I use almost daily to chill myself out is called abdominal breathing. This is basically breathing in and out using your tummy (abdominal) muscles instead of your chest. You take big, slow, deep breaths in and out through your nose, pushing your tummy in and out instead of moving your chest.

Breathing like this for about ten minutes will increase the supply of oxygen to your brain and stimulate the parasympathetic nervous system (the system responsible for relaxing your body), which promotes a state of calmness. Focusing on your breathing can also bring your awareness away from the worries in your head and will quieten your mind. Start doing it right now and feel the instant effect. Pretty cool.

LEARN TO SAY NO

This is another one I am really bad at! But there are a lot of advantages to learning to say no — or at least to taking the time to consider what you are being asked to do and whether you really need to or are capable of doing it. It's very easy to become conditioned to saying yes to every demand people make of you, especially if you want to get ahead at work or don't want to let employers, workmates and friends down. And then there's every 'yes' you give out in your personal life, including invitations to social events and other commitments, out of FOMO (fear of missing out). It can sometimes get to the point where all this fun stuff becomes stressful, and a chore, and you just need some time for yourself.

Don't be afraid to say no. It won't be the last time you get asked to do anything. You won't miss out on anything. At work saying no can sometimes be an advantage, if it gives you time to complete another task to a better standard, and people will respect you more for knowing your capabilities and ability to perform to expectations — both your own and your workmates'.

And don't feel like you have to explain yourself. If you want to say no to something, just say no. Then go ahead and use that time to complete other tasks, spend more time doing something else that you would rather do, or just enjoy the space you have just created in your busy life to relax and de-stress. And don't feel guilty or about it — you're doing this to maintain your mental health. You're doing a positive thing by looking after yourself. After all, if you don't look after yourself, you wont be able to look after anyone else.

STOP WORRYING AND REMIND YOURSELF WHAT'S GOOD

I know it's a cliché, but it's worth taking time out to appreciate the little things, even when the big things are getting you down. There will always be deadlines and other work pressures, and issues with family, friends or relationships to deal with. I think it is human nature to worry about these things, but getting caught up in these worries will consume you. The human brain has evolved to naturally think of worst-case scenarios in order to prepare us for them so we have the best chance of survival. This may have been useful back in hunter-gatherer times, when life-or-death situations were faced far more frequently, but today worries are perhaps the greatest misuse of the imagination. They are a waste of energy and thought, predominantly focused on things that will never eventuate.

We often ignore people who say to us, 'Don't worry about it,' but that really is the easiest way to save yourself the internal drama. The trick is finding ways to not worry. That is where I find it useful to change my train of thought and remind myself of all of the good things that are happening in my life, and in the lives of those who I care about — generally all the good things that surround us and we take for granted.

For me, one thing that always makes me feel good is to think about where we live.

We are simply so lucky here in New Zealand, and we need to appreciate that. We live in a country that is one of the safest in the world, and surely one of the most beautiful. I don't know of many other places that have mountains, forests, lakes, beaches and lush paddocks literally at your doorstep. In most New Zealand cities, no matter where you are, you are never more than a half-hour drive from a beach! Being in nature is so good for your mood, and never fails to lift my spirits.

Sometimes the stress and worries caused by work, relationships and other perceived problems feel as though they are holding your mind hostage, not wanting to release their grip and let you feel happy. This is when I find it helpful to focus on and appreciate all the other things that are going on around me. I find it good to socialise and spend time with other people, and get a bit of an insight into what's happening in their lives. It's easy to get caught up in your own stuff and forget that other people have stuff going on too — good and bad. My mum once said to me when I was growing up that 'everyone is going through shit'. Sure, it's not a very pretty quote, and Mum will probably be a little annoyed that, out of the countless pieces of wisdom she has shared with me over the years, this is what made it into this book! But it really rings true and I always carry this thought in the back of my mind, because you never know what other people are going through. We often get consumed in our own problems and forget that every single person in the world has their own 'shit' that they are going through.

Doing things for other people is another good way to keep your mental health ledger on the positive side. Quite interestingly, doing nice, positive, selfless things for others can be an almost selfish act in itself. But that's not a bad thing — you're just doing something that is going to make someone else feel good, knowing that it's going to make you feel good too! Win-win. And if you really get off on helping others then have a go at doing some volunteering — it can be a pretty cool feeling and it won't cost you a cent.

GOAL SETTING

I talked a bit about this in the exercise section (see chapter 17), but I think it's important to have goals and be working towards things you want to achieve in all aspects of your life, personal and professional.

Like your training and health goals, all your goals need to be achievable: there's no point in setting yourself up to fail. But don't make your goals too easy, either — that's not very satisfying. You want your goals

WHAT IF ITS NOT WORKING?

~~~

Your mental health is so crucial because it's what helps you to keep everything on track and achieve all the things you want to in life. Sometimes you try all these things and you still feel down. If you are eating well, exercising regularly and trying some of the suggestions here and it's still not helping, it's important you find something that does — and in some instances it's best to go straight to the pros. Seeking professional medical advice can help you to find out what's going on and how to make it better.

to be sufficiently challenging that you have to make some change or adaptation, or push yourself in some way to get there, but you also want to eventually succeed and feel good about what you have achieved.

Experts say you should write your goals down, along with a deadline of when you want to have achieved them by, then keep them somewhere you can see them so you stay motivated. I am not a particularly organised goal setter: I have goals but I don't write them down. As I mentioned before, one of my overall goals is to create the healthiest body I can, through nutrition and exercise. My other goals are often sub-goals leading to that overall goal. For example, at the time of writing I have the goal of training for and competing in Fight for Life, boxing against ex-All Black Zac Guildford. I have a goal to improve my core fitness and muscle endurance. From an aesthetic point of view, I want to maintain my current size and shape. Whatever your current fitness and exercise regime is, you're bound to have goals you want to work towards and achieve, whether a goal weight, body-fat percentage, number of reps, personal best time or whatever. And you can keep changing it up and challenging yourself to succeed.

In terms of my nutrition goals, every week my goal is the same: to eat as close to a paleo template as possible. It's like an ongoing challenge that I am happy to tick off each week. But, if you're just starting out down the paleo pathway, you'll be able to set yourself heaps of little goals and challenges: giving up sugar, cutting back on processed foods, going without bread, trying new paleo foods and so on.

When it comes to mental health I also have some goals. Firstly, I always try to get as close to eight hours of sleep a night as possible, because I know this has the greatest effect on my mental health. I also aim to do some form of exercise every day, be it a fitness class, a run or a walk, as I know that this makes me feel good and gives me a sense of accomplishment. I also try to achieve a couple of social events or interactions with friends every week, which takes my mind off any stress. I make an effort to talk to friends and catch up with family, to find out what's going on in their lives, see if I can help in any way and just to remind myself that my life is not any more important than anyone else's.

TIP: Routine can be a really good way of sticking to your goals and resolutions in terms of exercise and nutrition. Always exercising at the same time and making that an unbreakable appointment or making a rule to eat dinner at home every night during the week can really help you to stick to working on achieving your goals.

23. NOW IT'S UP TO YOU

So, there you have it. I said at the start of the book that I wanted to share with you my knowledge and experience of health, nutrition, fitness and wellbeing, and I think I have fulfilled that promise. As I have already mentioned many times, I truly believe that a paleo lifestyle is the best possible nutritional template for the human body. It has had such a large, positive impact on my health and my life in general that I urge you to give it a crack and experience some of these benefits for yourself.

I hope you have learnt some things about your body, how important your health is, and how to achieve that health. We have barely scratched the surface of this stuff, and I hope this book has encouraged you to look deeper into whatever aspects of nutrition and exercise interest you most. The more you learn about your body — both from reading and from experience — the more you can benefit your overall health, happiness and quality of life. Now it's your turn to eat clean and live lean.

FURTHER READING

.... •

Here are some books and websites which provide more information about the paleo lifestyle, functional fitness and other topics discussed in this book.

READ

Accidentally Overweight, Dr Libby Weaver (Little Green Frog Publishing Ltd, 2010)

Grain Brain, David Perlmutter with Kristin Loberg (Little, Brown and Company, 2013)

Luke and Scott: Clean Living, Scott Gooding and Luke Hines (Hachette Australia, 2013)

That Sugar Book, Damon Gameau (Pan Macmillan, 2014) — see also *That Sugar Film*, the original movie Gameau made

The Paleo Diet, Dr Loren Cordain (John Wiley & Sons, Inc., 2002, updated edition 2011)

The Paleo Diet for Athletes, Dr Loren Cordain (Rodale Books, 2005, updated edition 2012)

The Paleo Solution: The Original Human Diet, Robb Wolf (Victory Belt Publishing, 2010)

CLICK

clean-paleo.com

eatdrinkpaleo.com

lukeandscott.com

nomnompaleo.com

paleoleap.com

robbwolf.com — I really like this guy's style, not too sciency

tastypaleo.co.nz — recipes and a local café guide

thepaleodiet.com — the website of the original paleo guru, Dr Loren Cordain

WATCH

Eat, Fast and Live Longer — Dr Michael Mosley's documentary, available to watch online at vimeo.com/103656060

ACKNOWLEDGEMENTS

•••••••••••••••

This book is for my mum and dad, who have shaped me into the man I am today and who support me in whatever I do. For my sister, Emily, who always has my back and who inspires me to create. For my friends, who make me laugh and keep me smiling. And for Matilda, for her constant support and belief in me.

I want to thank all of the people at Allen & Unwin for helping me turn my thoughts into a book. Jenny, you helped me discover my love of writing. Sarah Ell, you're an amazing woman all round. Without all of your help this book would have been pretty shit, to be honest.

I also want to thank bananas, eggs and the guy who invented burpees.